Contents

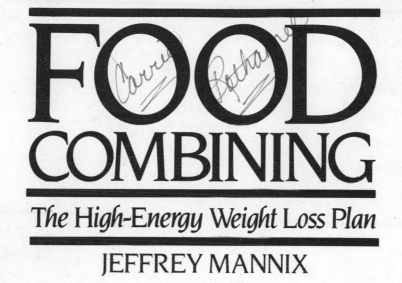

FOOD COMBINING

The High-Energy Weight Loss Plan

JEFFREY MANNIX

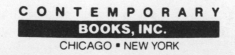

CONTEMPORARY
BOOKS, INC.
CHICAGO • NEW YORK

Library of Congress Cataloging-in-Publication Data

Mannix, Jeffrey.
    Food combining.

    Includes index.
    1. Nutrition.   2. Diet.   3. Health.   4. Longevity.
I. Title.
RA784.M35   1983   613.2   83-1879
ISBN 0-8092-5662-2
ISBN 0-8092-5661-4 (pbk.)

Published by Contemporary Books, Inc.
180 North Michigan Avenue, Chicago, Illinois 60601
Manufactured in the United States of America
Library of Congress Catalog Card Number: 83-1879
International Standard Book Number: 0-8092-5662-2 (cloth)
                                    0-8092-5661-4 (paper)

Published simultaneously in Canada by Beaverbooks, Ltd.
195 Allstate Parkway, Valleywood Business Park
Markham, Ontario L3R 4T8 Canada

Dedicated to Janice Morrissey of Ross, California for her wonderful skill and patience editing the original manuscript. And Pax Quigley for her support, encouragement, and love. And to all the volunteers, clients, and friends who faithfully contributed to the research.

Author's Foreword

Food combining is the result of the exhaustive research of an association of physicians practicing during the first quarter of the 20th Century, known as Hygenists.

The Hygenists saw the practice of medicine becoming more specialized after the turn of the century, and the use of drugs and surgery as primary treatment more accepted. Their concern was that the patient was becoming more and more partitioned in the eyes of the physician, and disease was being seen as localized problems of specific areas or functions of the body and unrelated to the individual as a whole. The Hygenists mounted an eloquent but futile campaign to remind the medical community of their responsibility to treat the patient as a whole person rather than merely the sum of many parts.

The Hygenists' holistic movement was trampled by progress, but the principles were carried on at the periphery of the medical establishment until the past ten years where they have surfaced again to gain the support of millions throughout the world who are realizing that every one of us is responsible for his own health, and that the only effective treatment for disease is prevention.

The Hygenists were accused of holding medical progress back by continuing to use fasting, hot baths, vitamin therapy, and bed rest to treat the body weakened by disease. Now, just fifty years later, the high cost of modern medical treatment along with the mediocre results of surgery and drug dependent methods are sending people back to basic sources of health care.

Thanks to the persistence of J. H. Tilden, Herbert Shelton, Otto Carque, and George Werger; the clear thinking of the entire Hygenic movement; Health Research in Molelumne Hill, California for preserving and republishing all the original Hygenist research; and to the "health nuts" for keeping the holistic movement alive, I am able to reintroduce food combining to the enormous number of people who are pursuing better health as a cure for disease.

The body will heal itself and become stronger if the environment within and surrounding is made agreeable. Achieving superior health is the medicine of the future. Food combining is one of the necessary prescriptions.

This book is offered to those who want to get better—feel better, look better, and live longer. I am convinced of the contribution food combining can make. It is now for you to discover.

My best wishes for your success.

Jeffrey Mannix
Los Angeles, California

1

Introduction

The information in this book is intended for people who want to know more about being healthy and living longer. It is dedicated to those people who want to achieve and maintain a sound mind and a body that works at peak efficiency. This book is for those individuals who have already enjoyed an acceptable level of well-being and are actively searching for higher levels of health, as well as those recovering from illness or pursuing better health for the first time.

This is not a diet book nor a compilation of prescriptions for relieving disease. Functional disorders of all kinds—overweight, headaches, arthritis, colitis, diabetes, hardening of the arteries, insomnia, ulcers, allergies, alcoholism, depression, hair loss, constipation, low energy, and myriad other symptoms of disorder are always manifestations of a chronic low level of total health.

The body is a complex and intricate machine with highly specialized systems. Despite the enormous scientific advances that have been made during this century, little progress has been made toward understanding the body's processing of food. So little investigation has been pursued, in fact, that health professionals have opted for becoming experts on disease. Specialists have chosen to excel in electronic diagnosis and chemical and surgical treatment of dysfunction in bodies that have been maintained inadequately. These treatments, which are usually temporary cures at best, are sometimes more detrimental than the dysfunctions or the disease they treat.

The selection and the combining of foods must be addressed seriously in order to improve the quality of life in an era that is saturated with stress, strain, and untold anxiety. Understanding the processes that the body uses to convert food into fuel for energy is as crucial as the selection and the quality of the food itself. Modern food processing, sophisticated farming, and almost instant systems of delivery provide extraordinary varieties of food for anyone not too distant from a city. We are living in a food century, which is a kind of mixed blessing. We are being poisoned slowly by the chemicals used in get-it-done-fast methods of production, not to mention the pesticides, the synthetic colors, and the preservatives used for longer shelf life. We are the victims of high technology and of big business. In addition, we ignore all the facts of the chemistry of digestion when we eat incompatible foods that inhibit, immobilize, and sometimes even destroy digestive processes.

All of life is a matter of relationships. Miscombinations of food tax the digestive organs and confuse the digestive juices. Ingesting incompatible foods that require different digestive procedures actually punishes the body, creating additional malfunction and wasting needed nutrients. Miscombinations of food inhibit the body's ability to filter waste and to eliminate toxins that cause high acidity in the blood and toxic disintegration.

WHAT FOOD COMBINING MEANS

Almost everyone has felt physical discomfort after some of those good old-fashioned Thanksgiving dinners. Of course you ate too much turkey, stuffing, potatoes, vegetables, salads, pies, nuts, fruits, and other goodies. But it was not just the amount of food that you gorged on that caused the problem. The physical discomfort really came from combining unlike foods that are incompatible because they require different digestive processes.

The theory of food combining is very simple. The logic is very overwhelming. For example, protein requires hydrochloric acid in the stomach for its digestion. Starch requires ptyalin. But hydrochloric acid *destroys* ptyalin. One need hardly say more. That delicious, healthy potato (starch) that you ate will sit around in your stomach, undigested, while the hydrochloric acid works on the protein that you ate. Food that is not broken down into its component parts quickly will putrefy in the warm bacterial environment of the stomach and will pass into the intestines, where nutrient absorption (or assimilation) takes place. But, again, nutrients are destroyed in food that putrefies. And food that putrefies in the digestive tract gives off toxins (poisons) that are then absorbed by the blood. These toxins contaminate everything in their environment while they paralyze the intestines, preventing them from eliminating waste. It is easy to see the implications of continually bombarding the body with inferior and destructive fuel. Not only will the digestive system be prohibited from functioning normally, but every cell in the body will be saturated with blood that carries destructive properties.

Elimination is a body function that is as vital to health as the proper assimilation of nutrients. Organic waste is loaded with poisons. Also, it is important to understand that the many processes of the body work efficiently within very small tolerances. There are 15 trillion cells in the body, each needing a supply of fuel to stay alive. Each of these cells produces toxic waste that must be eliminated. If this toxic waste is detained, the body systems can compensate for poisons for just so long before a condition of toxemia begins to enervate the cells and eventually the entire body.

Combining foods properly will begin to detoxify the body, and the detoxification will start after just a few days of good food combining. Food combining does not usually require the elimination of particular foods from the diet. Rather, food combining is concerned with the arrangement of the foods that are ingested.

Sick bodies have an overabundance of toxins in the blood resulting from the inadequate elimination of the waste products of metabolism. The blood system feeds and replenishes cells. Healthy people, those people without disease, have fewer toxins circulating through their cells. Healthy people feel good, adjust well, and live longer. Combining foods intelligently is one of the first steps in achieving better health. Why? Because proper food combining detoxifies the blood and thereby reduces body stress and the resultant enervation and disease.

Complete detoxification is probably an ideal state that is not possible to attain, just as the absolute of anything is impossible to reach. As the body ages, for instance, metabolism slows down and performs less efficiently in supplying fuel to cells and in eliminating waste. In theory, however, if these two processes, assimilation and elimination, were to work with no interference, we could live forever. Of course, *forever* is, again, in the realm of the impossible. But eliminating poisons to enhance the quality of life is most certainly a privilege that each person can enjoy.

PRINCIPLES OF FOOD COMBINING

Proper food combining is not a fad diet or a trendy manipulation of the things we eat. It should become a lifetime habit that will permit your body to work closer to its potential for being healthy. These are not rules to be followed to lose unwanted pounds or to rid yourself temporarily of digestive distress, though both weight loss and digestive comfort will often result. The purpose of proper food combining is to effect efficient use of food for fueling the body.

Different foods require different digestive juices to be changed into fuel. The most powerful enzymatic action is required for proteins. The protein enzymes destroy the enzymes required by starches and fruits, causing them to be delayed and to ferment. Fermentation produces poisons and the food in waiting becomes compacted. The body becomes full of gas, bloated, constipated, and downright miserable. These are a few of the body conditions that make for colon cancer and for fat production.

The following rules and categories of food will be the basic material for food combining. Begin now to compare your eating practices with those of food combining, and try making any changes that seem easy and natural. You will understand it all before too long, and be an authority before you finish the book.

FOOD COMBINING RULES

1. Eat similar foods together.
2. Eat no more than one concentrated protein at each meal.
3. Eat starches and protein at separate meals.
4. Eat fats and proteins at separate meals.
5. Eat sugars and proteins at separate meals.
6. Eat acids and proteins at separate meals.
7. Do not consume beverages during meals.
8. Drink milk alone or with acid fruit.
9. Eat starches and acid foods at separate meals.
10. Eat no more than one starch at each meal.
11. Eat starches and sugars at separate meals.
12. Eat fruit alone, especially melons.
13. Eat desserts alone (best combined or followed with green salad).

EATING RULES

To optimize the benefits from food combining, remember these rules for providing the proper environment for digestion:

1. Do not eat when tired or exhausted or immediately following hard work or exercise.
2. Do not eat under stress.
3. Do not eat when sick. Allow your body to free itself of disease.
4. Eat only when hungry but do not ignore hunger.
5. Chew everything, especially starch, 25 times before swallowing.
6. Eat in a peaceful, tranquil atmosphere.
7. After miscombining, either skip the next meal or eat only raw vegetables.
8. Eat four parts fruit and vegetables to one part protein and starch.
9. Eat more raw food, less cooked food.

EATING ADVICE

1. Any food is processed best when eaten by itself (monomeal).
2. Lemon or lime juice, vinegar, and other acids limit juices necessary to digest protein and/or starch. So, for now, omit these acids from salad dressings unless these salads are combined with vegetables.

FOOD CATEGORIES

Proteins Include: Meat, fish, poultry, cheese, eggs, dairy, nuts and seeds, beans.

Starches Include: Potatoes, grain products, beans, parsnips, pumpkins, squash, bananas, pasta.

Fats Include: Avocados, butter, cheese, cream, margarine, mayonnaise, nuts, oils, peanut butter.

Acids Include: Citrus, pineapple, strawberries, tomatoes, cranberries, vinegar.

TOXEMIA

In the healthy body, when nerve energy, or vitality, is normal, toxic waste is eliminated as fast as it evolves. Metabolism is the process of tissue building and rebuilding that includes anabolism, or cell building, and catabolism, or cell destruction. The destroyed cells are the waste products of the metabolic process. Broken-down tissue is highly toxic and destructive of healthy surrounding tissues. When the vital nerve energy of the cleansing system is overstimulated by trying to process unusual amounts of toxins, the body becomes enervated. The system must work longer and harder to do less and less. Elimination is delayed, and wastes are retained. Toxins going nowhere are accumulated until crisis occurs. Toxemic emergency can easily lead to disease, since anything that diminishes nerve energy can potentially cause disease producing.

There will be no disease if the body eliminates poisons efficiently—poisons that are produced within the body and/or are introduced from the environment. Germs do not cause disease. An enervated elimination system permits germs to attack cells that are soaked with toxins. Toxins must be accumulated beyond the toleration point to permit crises to take place. The whole organism then begins an insidious deterioration. Chronic disease symptoms begin to appear. Every chronic disease starts with toxemia and with toxemic crisis. These episodes are repeated until the organism actually changes. Body systems that are taxed, enervated, and toxemic have little power to resist infection.

The forces of disease are all around us. Some of us don't catch colds, flues, rashes, viruses, or cancers because our immune systems prohibit their taking root. But if you overstress that protection system, disease is highly likely to follow. The disease is not the cold, flu, or cancer; the disease is the chronic deterioration of the energy that fights off the germs that are ever present.

Eating too much food taxes the body systems. Miscombining foods taxes body systems. Confusing the digestive processes results in delayed digestion, fermentation, and putrefication of foods. Waste retention heralds disease and hastens death.

FOOD ADDICTION

Nurture (learned patterns of behavior) is as important as nature (heredity) in forming the individual. Fixed, learned patterns of behavior are called *habits*. Habits become more fixed as they are repeated over and over again. Both good and bad habits become dependable, comfortable friends in the quest for pleasure and security. And these familiar behavior patterns harbor the seeds for addiction.

We all have some understanding about addictions to alcohol and drugs. But food addiction is too common and socially proper to be examined with an eye to all of its destructive aspects. Many university studies and medical journals are now reporting that overeating is a behavior disorder very similar to the abuse of alcohol, drugs, caffeine, tobacco. The drug is the food, and the overeater becomes addicted to the excitement that food stimulates in the central nervous system. Concentrated foods such as starch, meat, cheese, and sugar, cause the most excitement and are the most addicting. Miscombining foods also seems to produce an excitement from the toxins it produces. Eventually body tolerance develops, combined with a psychological need for the pleasurable substance. Then, more of the same becomes necessary to produce that good feeling. Poisons then tax the cells, resulting in chronic toxemia. If the causes of toxemia are not eliminated, disease will manifest itself through the body's weakest parts. Dysfunction, deterioration, even cancer, take over.

Balanced meals include everything under the sun. The digestive system is bombarded with protein, starch, vegetables, fruit, often sugar, and alcohol. We accept the custom of relaxing at day's end with some kind of alcohol even before we start the balanced meal. Most people in our culture have practiced these eating patterns long enough to feel comforted by them and happy with them. It is quite reasonable to say that most people are addicted to these eating habits. They are addicted to the enervating poisons that incompatible food combinations produce. They grow accustomed to poor health, to feeling less than well, to being bloated, sluggish, flatulent, constipated, toxic, and angry. Health, everyone's health, will improve when foods are combined intelligently. And everyone's health will improve when food is taken in moderation. The key words are *assimilation, elimination,* and *moderation.*

2

How Food Combining Works

UNDERSTANDING DIGESTION

In order to make food combining a significant part of your life, you must have a fundamental understanding of how the digestive process works. Knowing about the mechanics of digestion and elimination will illustrate the simple truth about food combining and will make you an expert at achieving your maximum health potential.

No doctor, hospital, or diagnostic machine can tell you more about your state of health than you can, and nothing contributes to your condition more directly than your digestive process. Life is not possible without food, and health is not possible without a system for changing food into the nutrient, vitamin, and mineral fuel that keeps the body growing and free of disease.

A clean-running, efficient digestive system is the key to superior health and long life. A poorly working digestive system is the cause of disease and death, no matter where the disease strikes or at what age death comes.

Take time to read this chapter carefully and to understand the mechanics of life. Food combining is based only on helping these functions work better.

THE MECHANICS OF DIGESTION

Digestion begins in the mouth. In the process of chewing, food is mixed with saliva and made soft. Saliva is 98-percent water and contains a mucous that gives it a sticky, syrupy consistency. Saliva also contains the enzyme ptyalin, which is needed to begin the process of digestion for starch foods in the mouth. Saliva is secreted by three pairs of glands that produce about a quart of saliva a day.

After food is chewed and mixed with saliva it is ready to be swallowed. The voluntary part of digestion ends there; the rest is automatic. The food is prevented from returning to the mouth by the back of the tongue and is forced into the esophagus, which is 10 inches long and less than an inch wide. It passes through the diaphragm and leads into the stomach.

The esophagus dilates and contracts over and over again until the food travels its length. This precisely timed contracting and relaxing of muscles is called *peristalsis,* and it permits food to travel to the stomach even while you are standing on your head.

The stomach is the largest, most muscular section of the digestive tract. When empty, it is J-shaped, with its top pressing against the diaphragm. When full, the stomach becomes pear-shaped. The capacity of the adult stomach is a little more than a quart and a half and will commonly hold some food for three or four hours before moving it ahead to the small intestine.

When food is held in the stomach it is churned and mixed with digestive juices. Because of the gas that is usually trapped in the stomach, be it full or empty, the churning of food often causes the rumbling that is sometimes embarrassingly audible. This gas also produces hunger pangs as it presses against the walls of an empty stomach.

The inner lining of the stomach is a mucous membrane that houses some 30 or 40 million glands that secrete the gastric enzymes called *digestive juice*. Digestive juice is a strong acid secretion that actually contains hydrochloric acid in varying amounts according to the nature of the food in the stomach. When digestion is poor acidity can become higher than usual and can cause more gas than is normal. Gas pushing against the walls of the stomach causes pain and, in trying to escape, can sometimes be forced up into the esophagus. Millions of dollars are made on the remedies for this condition that is familiarly called *heartburn*.

The walls of the stomach are protected from the acid secreted by its own glands by producing a mucous covering that protects it. When too much acid is produced regularly, portions of this mucous protection may be etched to allow the acid to contact the stomach tissue itself. The result is a gastric ulcer, believed to be caused by hyperacidity due to tension.

The pyloric sphincter at the lower end of the stomach stays tightly closed until the majority of the food in the stomach has been reduced to a liquid known as *chyme*. It then relaxes, and the peristaltic action of the stomach squeezes the chyme out into the intestines.

The intestines are divided into two segments: the first is a section approximately 25 feet long, known as the small intestine; final digestion and nutrient absorption take place here. The large intestine, about five feet long, is where water is absorbed from the waste matter about to be eliminated. The descriptions *small* and *large* refer to the width of the segments, not to the length.

The first part of the small intestine is the duodenum, a small section that is designed to receive the highly acid chyme mixture that comes from the stomach and to neutralize the acid before the chyme moves on to the more fragile part of the small intestine to be broken down further and then to be absorbed. The neutralizing juices come from the pancreas and the liver.

The pancreas is the second-largest gland in the body. It produces insulin to control blood sugar levels in one section and secretes a variety of digestive enzymes from another section. They include starch-splitting enzymes called *amylase* that continues the work begun by ptyalin in the mouth; a fat-splitting enzyme, called *lipase;* and several protein-splitting enzymes, among them trypsin and chymotrypsin, which continue the work begun by pepsin in the stomach.

Most digestion and all absorption of nutrients take place in the small intestine. The secretion from the liver that neutralizes the acidity in the duodenum is called *gall,* a yellow bile. Between meals some of the bile is stored in a pear-shaped sac beneath the right lobe of the liver called the *gallbladder*. Gall bile contains no enzymes for digestion. It has properties called *bile salts* that act as a detergent to neutralize acid and to emulsify fats into water-soluble units that will be compatible with the predominantly water-soluble enzymes. During this emulsifying action in the duodenum the yellow-green pigment of the bile colors the food, and this color stays with the food throughout the rest of the travel in the small and large intestines and is responsible for the color of the final waste product. Some of the pigment is also absorbed into the blood and gives both plasma and urine their amber color. As the nutrient-enriched blood moves from the liver into the capillaries of the tissues, the cells of the body absorb the glucose for energy and assimilate the protein for their own individual needs. Between meals, when new glucose is not being supplied from the small intestines, the liver draws on its store of glycogen, converting it again to glucose and slowly dripping it into the blood to be used as energy fuel. The liver has about 20 hours of glucose fuel stored as glycogen, after which the body will convert fat into glucose.

Fat collected in the small intestine that isn't used as a lubricant throughout the body or is not burned for heat is stored in the cells of a special connective tissue called *adipose tissue,* which is under the skin and insulates the body from extreme temperatures. It also settles around the organs to protect them from being jarred.

Slabs of adipose tissue protect the abdomen and the kidneys. These blankets of adipose tissue protect those organs that lie close to the surface from damaging injury, and they collect fat readily. These slabs are usually the first places to notice excess fat storage, but be aware of the fact that every other hidden space has been fatted before these areas.

Food takes approximately three hours to travel through the small intestine while being digested and absorbed. Digestion is completed when food is passed into the *colon*, which is part of the large intestine. The small intestine joins the large intestine at the lower right side of the body near the groin. The last six-inch section is called the *rectum,* and the opening to the outside is the *anus,* which is held tightly shut by the anal sphincter.

The function of the large intestine is to absorb water from the waste and then to eliminate the waste. As water is subtracted, the remains become more solid. The solid contents at the end of this long digestive process constitute the feces, which are composed of all the undigested elements of food. The act of eliminating the feces is called *defecation* and is accomplished by the peristaltic action of the rectum with abdominal muscle contraction.

The more roughage that is derived from indigestible plant cellulose, bran from grain coverings, and fiber from fruits and vegetables, the better is the peristaltic action of the large intestine, since it adds bulk and prohibits compacting of the waste material. Thus constipation is retained dehydrated and compacted feces. Diarrhea is just the opposite.

You should now have a basic grasp of the mechanics of digestion. Without interference the process will run smoothly and efficiently through the stages of digestion, absorption, and elimination. When interfered with, however, the process will adapt to get the jobs done by draining vital energy from the body. Whenever this system runs smoothly health will eventually improve, thinking will become clearer, and life will become better.

The Role of Enzymes

The complicated machinery of digestion depends on the chemical changes that affect the food within the system. The chemicals that are responsible for the disintegration of the basic elements from the foodstuff are called *enzymes.* Enzymes are catalysts. They are independent substances that make something happen to another substance without adding anything of themselves to the change or being in any way part of the reaction. Enzymes work very specifically. The body produces hundreds of enzymes, each a catalyst for one particular function. Within the digestive system a number of major enzymes have been identified, along with the specific classes of food substance that each acts on.

Digestion begins in the mouth, where food is broken into smaller particles and saturated with saliva. Most foods, however, are not subjected to the actions of enzymes until they have reached the stomach. Starch, however, is an exception. Saliva is an alkaline fluid that contains the enzyme ptyalin, which is the catalyst for breaking down starch into a simpler form called *maltose*. Starch must be converted to maltose to be ready for the next enzyme, maltase, which is found in the small intestine and turns the maltose into an even simpler form known as *dextrose*. (Starch is not digested in the stomach, there are no stomach or gastric enzymes specific to starch.) Maltase can only act specifically on maltose, not starch. Starch that escapes the effect of ptyalin in the mouth, and consequently cannot be acted on by maltase in the intestine, has one more chance to be broken down in the intestine. This is done by the pancreatic enzyme *amylase,* provided that the starch has not already begun to ferment in the warm incubating environment of the stomach.

Ptyalin can act only in an alkaline solution. A small trace of acid not only prevents the action of ptyalin but may also destroy the enzyme entirely. It is this limitation of the enzyme that makes the environment we set for it so important. If we mix starch with foods that are acid or that require acid secretion in the stomach, ptyalin will be destroyed, and starch digestion will stop. Starch that sits in a warm, moist, bacterial enclosure will ferment and will produce toxic gases almost immediately.

Stomach or gastric juice contains a number of enzymes, the most important of which is pepsin, which begins the digestion of all proteins. Pepsin is formed in the stomach and requires an acid environment not only to act on protein but for its very existence as well. Pepsin converts proteins into proteoses, peptones, and peptides in the stomach, which then pass on to the small intestine to be broken down further into amino acids by intestinal and pancreatic enzymes. The enzymes of the intestine and pancreas do not act on complex protein that has not been broken down; they act only on peptones and peptides. Without prior action of pepsin on the protein in the stomach, protein digestion would be incomplete. Pepsin is destroyed in an alkaline medium, by low temperature from cold drinks, and by high temperature from hot drinks and fever.

When the chyme leaves the stomach for the small intestine the pancreas combines with the liver to produce bile to neutralize the acid and contribute four very important digestive enzymes. Pancreatic anylase completes the digestion of starch, which was begun in the mouth; pancreatic lipase breaks down fats; pancreatic rennin continues the work of the gastric rennin in coagulating milk, thereby segregating the solids; and trypsin breaks down protein. The important thing to know about the pancreatic enzymes is that the most important one, trypsin, is destroyed by acid. If the bile is unable to neutralize the contents of the stomach, continued protein digestion may be impossible. Hyperacidity due to tension or illness of food fermenting because of bad food combinations may produce too much acid in the stomach for the bile to neutralize.

The final group of enzymes is manufactured in the small intestine and works on the simple compounds produced by the preceding enzymes to make them ready for absorption. Erepsin breaks out the final amino acids from polypeptides, and sucrase, maltase, and lactase make the final carbohydrate conversion into glucose.

Normal Digestion

The blood should receive amino acids for cell repair, simple sugar for energy, fatty acids and glycerol for heat and lubrication, vitamins and minerals to regulate metabolism, and water for electrical balance and the formation of tissue. Foods must be digested to be transformed into these necessities. Rotted, undigested food produces poison.

Anything that reduces digestive efficiency in any way that interferes with the precise timing of digestive enzymes will limit the nutrient end products of digestion and will increase the gaseous bacterial poisons absorbed by the blood. Damage to the body may not be dramatic with each episode, and some of us have even grown so accustomed to faulty digestion that we consider an occasional bout inevitable, as evidence by the over-the-counter antacid remedies that dominate pharmacy shelves. But cancer of the colon and of the stomach are still our biggest killers.

Ptyalin requires an alkaline medium in order to prepare starch for final digestion in the intestine. Ptyalin is destroyed by only a trace of acid. Pepsin requires an acid medium in the stomach to begin the digestion of protein. If meat and potatoes are combined at the same meal, the hydrochloric acid in the stomach will destroy the ptyalin and will end starch digestion. Undigested starch is absorbent and will readily absorb pepsin and slow the digestion of the protein. While the potato may have only required two hours in the stomach before leaving for the small intestine to finish the major part of its digestion, it must now wait five to six hours for the meat to finish the major part of its digestion in the stomach. The stomach environment is warm and moist. It is a haven for bacteria. Starch ferments easily, and without the benefit of enzymatic action it will definitely putrefy.

The stomach is a receptacle that is designed to decompose organic matter. If the appropriate enzymes are present, this decomposition is orderly and accomplished without side effects. However, if the catalysts are missing or are ineffective, the environment of the stomach promotes deterioration.

In the final analysis, combining foods that have competing digestive needs inevitably assigns one or both to destruction in the stomach. The results are always uncomfortable and eventually damaging. Physicians report that complaints of gas and stomach bloating are among the most common medical ailments they treat. Couple that with the overwhelmingly high incidence of digestive cancer, it appears obvious that there is something very wrong with either what or how we are eating.

Food combining is really an enzyme-matching process. How sad it is to select fresh, high-quality food and then have it rot within our bodies because we are not prepared to receive it. Be prepared. There are only a few categories of food. Know their digestive requirements and achieve your full potential.

Protein is digested in the stomach with acid. It stays in the stomach for from three to six hours, longer if mixed with starch. It can produce the most toxic waste.

Starch is digested in the small intestine. The first stage begins in the mouth. It must be chewed thoroughly and mixed with saliva, which contains ptyalin. Digestion is stopped by acid. Starch ferments quickly if digestion is delayed, which then causes gas and constipation.

Fruit is the most easily digested food. It leaves the stomach rapidly. It ferments easily, so eat it alone, and never combine it with protein or starch. Fruit will turn to alcohol and contaminate foods that need time in the stomach for digestion.

Fat combines well with starch. Both are digested in the small intestine. Fat retards protein digestion.

Stress Digestion

To ensure a rich and steady flow of enzymes to the foods we eat, we must be aware of a few things.

Chewing starts the entire digestive process. Food can be identified in the mouth when it is adequately chewed, and the right enzymes will begin secreting into the stomach in preparation to receive it. Deliberately chewing all food until it is pastelike will unburden the digestive system and put that much less stress on the body.

Minimizing stress on the body is the ultimate goal of food combining. Efficiency of operation without unnecessary effort keeps a machine running best and longest. Many health researchers now agree that there is no disease that is not stress related, and by the same token, health is enhanced by eliminating stress. Stress on the digestive system will be eliminated by proper food combining. More stress can be alleviated at the same time if you follow the rule of never eating when you feel tense.

Eating when you are nervous, anxious, angry, fearful, or upset promotes overacid indigestion of the food you eat. Eating when chilled or overheated, feverish, in pain, fatigued, or just before or after work overtaxes an already overtaxed body.

The more tension that you bring to eating, the more ineffective digestion will be, and the larger your problem becomes. Perastalsis is paralyzed by tension, and food then moves slower through the system. The stomach and the saliva become too acidic, and the secretion of enzymes is curtailed or prohibited. Food is not digested completely or eliminated properly. Tension is compounded, with more stress resulting. Eventually something must give. The most identifiable crises of stress are: stroke, heart attack, ulcers, nervous breakdown. Eliminate stress in your life! Food combining will contribute largely if you come to the table in peace.

3

Results of Food Combining

THE KEY TO HEALTH

Stress comes from many areas of life, not just the emotional. Food combining helps eliminate physical stress by streamlining the digestive process to produce less toxin and poisonous waste matter. Stress reduction contributes one key element in promoting health—alkalinity of the blood.

Medicine has always recognized that a high acid level of the blood, referred to as acidosis, is a dangerous imbalance that can result in death if allowed to persist.

The blood is naturally alkaline unless it is influenced to become acid. Acid formers are the stresses of tension, lack of sleep, alcohol, tobacco, caffeine, natural toxins from the digestive system, and the highly poisonous waste product of normal cell replacement. Stress produces acid in the blood, and the pursuit of superior health must attempt to eliminate as much of this acid as possible.

Certain foods, just from their mineral composition, are acid-forming. The second level of food combining will prepare you to recognize acid-forming foods and counterbalance them with foods whose mineral composition are alkaline forming.

THE ALKALINE BALANCE

As food influences the blood, two things can be done to maintain a high level of alkalinity in the blood:

1. Combine foods in the proper way so that they won't cause fermentation, incomplete digestion, or acid-forming toxins.

2. Complement all acid-forming foods with foods containing significant amounts of alkaline elements to keep the alkaline balance in the blood high.

To keep the alkaline balance strong, just be careful not to mix protein foods with starch foods, sugar with starch, acid with starch, or fruit with anything. You will become more sophisticated with food combining as you learn and as you experience the rewards of this practice.

Alkaline-forming foods include all vegetables, especially if they are eaten raw; all fruit; and raw milk and raw milk products.

The acid-forming foods are flesh foods; eggs; cheese; cereals and cereal products; legumes; the peanut, filbert and Brazil nut; all roasted nuts; sulphur-treated fruits and fruits preserved in syrup; refined sugar; candy; chocolate; cocoa; butter; margarine; lard and hydrogenated oils; coffee; tea; artificially sweetened drinks, and alcohol.

The rule for offsetting the acid-forming foods is to eat four alkaline foods for every acid-forming food. In other words, 80 percent of the diet should be fruit, vegetables and raw dairy products, with 20 percent being proteins, cereals, legumes, etc. Seventy-five percent of alkaline fruits and vegetables should be raw, since high heat used to process food destroys alkalinity.

HOW ACID FORMS

The process of tissue building in the body is called *metabolism*. Within metabolism there is cell building, called *anabolism*, and cell destruction, called *catabolism*. All the cells in the body are continually wearing out and being replaced. Worn-out cells are replaced a little at a time, and we must eat foods containing protein to supply the raw material for building. The cast-off parts of the cells are oxidized protein, which is highly acid-forming nitrogen and is ever so slightly poisonous, or toxic. The circulating blood transfers this broken-down tissue to the liver, kidneys, and lungs to be eliminated. In a healthy system the dead tissue is cleaned from the cells by the blood as quickly as it is evolved and then filtered out of the blood and eliminated from the body without delay.

The toxic waste of catabolism is not the only acid that enters the blood for immediate elimination. The end products of the digestion of certain foods picked up by the blood are acid-forming once they are burned and must be eliminated just as urgently.

Acids that are not part of the necessary working of the body can also enter the blood. For instance, tobacco is acid-forming, as are alcohol, coffee, and tea. Drugs make the blood acidic, as do pain, fear, anger, worry, and fatigue. And one of the largest contributors of unnecessary acid to the body is the bacterial fermentation of food in the digestive tract.

At some point the toxins circulating in the blood will increase while waiting for elimination. The cells retain waste and are then delivered more waste. Toxins that were relatively harmless as long as they were neutralized and eliminated as quickly as they were produced now band together into waves of poisons. More of the cell dies than is normal and is replenished with inferior material. This condition is known as *toxemia*. It is the beginning of all disease, and once it is established, it will continue until the causes of the overloading are removed or until the body falls prey to disease.

TOXEMIA

Disease is caused by weakened health from the retention of too much waste for too long. Disease is a violent way for the body to cleanse itself of the acid waste infecting all the cells of all tissue. The crisis just happens to appear at the weakest spot in the body. Cancer, heart disease, or rheumatism are not just bad luck. They took hold in systems that were forced to handle too many poisons for too long. They began as recurring headaches, bleeding gums, frequent colds, or a nagging cough—all warnings, local symptons of general disorder.

It follows that it is futile to try to cure the headache, or bleeding gums, allergies, or hemorrhoids. The body is trying to eliminate poisons that are irritating and choking every cell. The normal steps of elimination have been unable to handle the load for a long time until one of the crises was established. The poisons must be let out. If they are masked with drugs, toxemia will continue to get worse until the causes of the buildup of the waste are eliminated or a critical function of the body collapses.

STIMULANTS

The use of stimulants—alcohol, tobacco, coffee, tea, cocoa, sugar, narcotics, and food—contributes more acid to the blood than any other outside source, and with their potential for addiction they must be considered lethal. If the use of any of these stimulants becomes a habit, you can be sure that you are becoming enervated and toxemic.

Stimulants rob the body of its alkalinity and elicit the flow of adrenaline and other hormones that temporarily increase energy and excite the mind. But the energy that stimulants provide is received at the expense of the vital energy of the entire body and must be paid back with interest. Fooling the body to produce energy that it wouldn't normally produce overtaxes the very core of the system. When the stimulant has run its course and the borrowed energy has been expended, painful recuperation is necessary. The pain may be postponed, however, by turning again to the stimulant—and again and again. Addiction has you in its clutches before you know it.

Food is a stimulant, and the acid-forming foods behave in the very same way as other, better known drugs. The acid-forming proteins and starches are slightly poisonous to the system, and the body reacts by increasing the heart rate, flushing the blood with adrenaline, and becoming generally aroused. Constant overuse will slowly develop dependence and eventual trouble.

Overweight people have been trapped by the addiction to stimulating food. They have developed eating habits that are out of their control because they use food to elevate their mood and have become addicted to the slow poisoning.

Approach stimulating foods such as proteins, starch, and sugar with caution. Exclude all acid-forming food from at least one meal every day to keep a safe distance from being trapped.

MINERAL ELEMENTS

Minerals, also known as organic salts, are the elements within all foods that give each food its acid-forming or alkaline character.

The organic salts come from the soil, sun, air, and water and are supplied to us directly or indirectly from plants. They enter the body as fully oxidized compounds, furnishing practically no heat or energy. They need no processing, as proteins and starches do; they are directly useful to the body, since they are provided from the plant source.

Although minerals make up only 5 percent of the body, they are absolutely essential to life. They provide the nerves with a vital electricity and magnetism that keep electrical pathways charged and juices flowing. Minerals are responsible for cells maintaining their firmness and form. They regulate absorption through the cell walls by making osmosis possible; they attract waste in the blood and help remove it; they carry oxygen and give a vital resistance to every cell, making the body invulnerable to infection from the outside.

The acid-forming mineral elements are: phosphorus, sulphur, silicon, chlorine, fluorine, iodine, and arsenic. The acid-binding (alkaline) elements are: potassium, sodium, calcium, magnesium, iron, manganese, and aluminum.

It is perhaps the opposing forces of acid forming and acid

binding that charge the minerals with their vital electric forces that hold our cells firm and promote the push-pull of osmosis. All the mineral elements are necessary, but some have a reputation for being more necessary them others, such as iron, potassium, and calcium. Since only a very small amount of any mineral is needed, all the minerals can be supplied adequately if a raw vegetable salad is eaten every day.

SUPPLEMENTS

There is no doubt that the body can absorb vitamins and minerals in a processed and condensed form. There are people who say that they owe their lives to vitamin and mineral pills. And there are physicians who cure disease symptoms with massive doses of vitamins and minerals and psychiatrists who cure the most bizarre emotional disorders with the use of megadoses of vitamins and minerals. It seems quite possible that vitamin and mineral supplements can help restore balance to a system that is enervated and failing. A relaxing day in the sun, a hot bath, some time in a steam room, or a massage would also help. For healthy people who maintain their fitness, commercially prepared supplements may become a burden, possibly adding more toxins that will need to be eliminated.

Mineral elements may be combined and packaged in various combinations, but after they are swallowed and digested it isn't known how, or whether, they are used. All that is really known for sure is that the liver and kidneys are overworked trying to eliminate them.

How can minerals keep the cells charged with the spark of life coming from the dried, pulverized, lifeless form of a pill? A vitamin C capsule containing 1,000 milligrams of vitamin concentrate cannot be the same as the 15 oranges it was extracted from. The life is gone, and maybe that unexplainable "life" is the very thing that we need from the vitamin source and not the stuff that can be extracted.

It seems that the vitamin industry has intimidated the public into buying expensive supplements based on the diagnosis of people with disease. In analyzing disease, they project findings to those who enjoy good health. The logic is deceptive.

Vitamins and minerals come from plants before they come from any other source. Each time they are processed, either by an animal or by a machine, they lose some of their vitality. As in the processing and refining of food, eventually the only thing left is the most basic ingredient. White bread, for instance, is not able to support life, though analysis shows that it contains starch, protein, vitamins, and minerals in the same proportion as the grain from which it was made.

Get your vitamins and minerals from uncooked fruits and vegetables. And if you neglect your diet and exercise, turn to the supplements with a prayer.

4

Protein Combinations

WHAT PROTEINS ARE

Next to water, protein is the most abundant ingredient in the body. Protein is never absent from the protoplasm of any living tissue, animal or vegetable, and is vitally connected with every expression of organic activity. Protein is the primary source of building material for the blood, muscles, skin, hair, nails, internal organs, and brain, as well as for cell replacement.

Protein is also necessary for the formation of hormones, which control body function, and for enzymes, which regulate metabolism. Hemoglobin, the critical oxygen-carrying molecule of the blood, is a protein. Protein in the blood helps regulate the body's water balance and aids in clotting. In addition, protein is necessary for the formation of antibodies to fight bacterial and viral infection.

Protein is so indispensable in the building and functioning of the body that we may think of ourselves as made up of protein. Protein is a highly complex compound of carbon, hydrogen, nitrogen, oxygen, and sulphur and exists in a solid, semisolid, or liquid state in nearly all of the solids and liquids of the body.

In plants the protein is composed of simple chemical compounds derived directly from the minerals in the soil. In animals this synthesis cannot occur, so protein must come directly or indirectly from vegetables.

AMINO ACIDS

During digestion protein is broken down into smaller component parts called *amino acids,* which the body needs for the construction of human protein. The amount of amino acid in that food determines its quality.

The body requires 22 amino acids in a specific pattern to make human protein. Fourteen of these can be produced within the body, and the eight that must come from outside sources must be supplied simultaneously in proportions corresponding to those existing in the body in order to carry out protein synthesis. The eight amino acids that the body requires from food sources are called *essential amino acids.* If just one essential amino acid is missing, protein synthesis will fall to a very low level or stop completely. If all the essential amino acids are present, but one is of low strength, it is believed that all of the amino acids will be reduced to the strength level of the weak one. This weak one is called the *limiting amino acid,* and the strength of this weakest amino acid determines the biological value of protein food.

When a food contains all the essential amino acids, it is called a *complete protein.* Foods that are extremely low in or lack one of the eight essential amino acids are incomplete proteins and therefore must be considered insufficient for the body's protein requirement. To be useful they must be fortified with another protein food that has a plentiful amount of the limited amino acid.

METABOLIZING PROTEIN

Before any food can be used as fuel for the body it must be processed through the various stages of digestion. Again, digestion begins in the mouth, where foods are broken up into smaller particles by chewing before being passed into the stomach, where gastric juices chemically disintegrate them and make them ready for the final stages of digestion and for the absorption that takes place in the intestines. During the chewing process the type of food is identified, and the appropriate enzymes are added to the saliva and also begin to secrete into the stomach.

Remember that each enzyme is very specific, acting only on one class of food substance during any of the various stages of digestion. Each stage requires different enzymes, and each enzyme can be effective only if the preceding work has been done by the preceding enzyme. If, for example, conflicting enzymes are needed at the same time, the strongest one will dominate and will prevent the weaker enzyme from processing the other food, leaving it to decompose and to turn into toxic waste.

Protein digestion requires an acid environment in the stomach and establishes this environment with an outpouring of hydrochloric acid in a concentration that depends on the character of the protein that was eaten.

In the acid environment of the stomach the enzyme pepsin initiates the digestion of all types of protein. Pepsin acts on complex protein, breaking it down into peptones. These components of protein then are split into amino acids. Without the prior action of pepsin to reduce protein to peptones, the other enzymes would not act on the protein, amino acids would not be broken out, and even the highest-quality protein would not be utilized and would be wasted.

Extra acid produced by fear, anger, anxiety, exhaustion, or illness or consumed in the form of citrus juice, vinegar, mustard, tomatoes, or other acids used in food preparation suspends the secretion of hydrochloric acid and interferes with the work of pepsin in the digestion of protein. An alkaline environment in the stomach also interferes with the action of pepsin, thus making the protein/starch combination especially poor.

DIFFERENCES IN PROTEINS

All foods contain some protein, some with a high amount of

the essential amino acids, but many with low strengths of the eight essential amino acids. In the selection of protein, attention must be paid to choosing protein foods that will supply all the essential amino acids at the same meal. Although research in nutrition has always yielded inadequate information on how the body metabolizes food, it is believed that all the essential amino acids must be present at the same meal in order to supply useful protein to the body. It is therefore necessary to choose protein foods that contain all the essential amino acids or to select carefully the foods that will complement each other to make complete usable protein.

USABLE PROTEIN

Be aware of the fact that the measured amount of protein in any food is never equal to the amount of protein that the body can use from that food. Usable protein is different with each food, determined by the weakest amino acid of the essential amino acids found in that food. It is much like a chain being as strong as its weakest link. So, it is from the limiting amino acid in a protein food that we must measure the amount of available protein and, from that measure, determine the usable protein and then how much we need.

Also keep in mind that some protein foods may contain so many calories and/or acid-forming elements that they may not really be the best source of protein. Perhaps twice the amount of another protein food with half the amount of usable protein may prove to be a better choice.

Learn enough about protein to make daily selections that will supply your protein needs without taxing the digestive process. By combining foods properly, all protein will be made more usable for the body. Even protein foods that may be considered lower in quality because of weak essential amino acids will supply more of their usable protein.

It is safe to assume that between 10 and 35 percent of animal protein is unusable despite digestion and that between 30 and 60 percent of the protein in vegetable sources is unusable. The following table will give you a working knowledge of the usable protein available in the major food groups.

Protein Food	Usable Amount
Eggs	94%
Milk	82%
Yogurt	82%
Fish	80%
Cottage cheese	75%
Rice	70%
Swiss cheese	70%
Tofu (soybeans)	65%
Meat/chicken	65%
Grains	55%
Nuts	50%
Vegetables	60%

When considering protein, four factors must be evaluated:

1. _Quality._ Protein of low quality must be teamed with other protein to strengthen the weak amino acids.

2. _Amount._ Two ounces of concentrated high-quality protein food will supply the entire daily requirement; more food is necessary with low-quality sources.

3. _Acidity._ Most protein foods are acid-forming in varying degrees. Knowing this will indicate food combinations for keeping acid levels down.

4. _Clogging Effect._ Portions of all foods will go undigested. Know if this residue will sweep (cleanse) or clog the system.

With some care you will be able to select usable protein that will not only supply all the essential amino acids but will also provide necessary roughage without overloading the system with acid waste.

ANIMAL PROTEIN

Flesh Foods

While there are slight differences in the amounts of usable

protein found in meat, fish, and poultry, flesh foods provide all the essential amino acids in very concentrated form. Expect to be supplied with between 60 and 80 percent of usable protein in all flesh foods. Because of this high concentration, fiber or roughage is missing entirely from this kind of protein, and it is therefore considered easily digestible. The average time for the digestion of flesh foods, barring digestive interference, is four hours.

But flesh foods, containing no fiber, should be combined with liberal amounts of vegetables in order to supply the fibrous roughage that is so critical to the intestines and to counterbalance high acidity. And be aware of the fact that meat is by no means essential to health.

In the muscular tissues of a dead animal the lifegiving forces are in the process of decline. They have been lost in the production of animal heat, energy, electricity, and body function. And, as discussed earlier, animal tissue replacement and growth means deterioration and toxic waste production. The vitality of animal tissue depends on continuous removal of waste poisons. Stalled poisons accelerate the decomposition of flesh.

Flesh proteins are thus less nutritional than plant proteins because flesh foods contain, along with their protein, a concentration of poisons, which are found in the tissues of all animals. It makes little sense to eat foods that contain the very poisons we try to eliminate when we combine foods intelligently.

Evidence suggests that man is primarily a fruit- and nut-eating animal and that only recently in his evolution has he turned to eating meat, and perhaps even grain only out of necessity. Carnivorous animals have atrophied, inactive sweat glands, whereas man, and other fruit-eating and vegetable-eating animals, have well-developed sweat glands. These glands were retained by carnivores as rudimentary organs, like the appendix in man, but the sweat glands have completely lost their function of sweating. This protects the carnivore against loss of water through the skin and consequently leads to retention of waste poison in the system. Uric acid, one of the most lethal waste products of metabolism, is produced in abundance after the digestion of meat. Uric acid dissolves in warm water and can be kept circulating in the blood of the carnivore as long as an adequate amount of water is retained. Inactive sweat glands in the carnivore assure the circulation of uric acid, but when the animal dies the uric acid settles in the muscles and organs and quickly sours the tissues. It follows that since man is subject to sweating, it is evident that he was not intended to live on flesh and other highly acid-forming foods. The accumulation of uric acid in the system can be the cause of gout, rheumatism, kidney disease, hardening of the arteries, high blood pressure, heart disease, liver disease, and nervous disorders.

Flesh foods have a kind of stimulating effect, largely due to the amount of waste poison they contain. Circulation is increased after the ingestion of flesh foods in order to eliminate the toxins it contains, producing the temporary illusion of vitality. This additional "borrowed energy" is short-lived and is followed by weakness, nervousness, and enervation. The next time you eat a flesh meal, carefully examine the effects it has on your energy. Notice your elevated heart rate and how quickly this borrowed energy has to be paid back after the meal.

In the plant kingdom life forces are ascending and act beneficially on the functions of the body. Plants are constructive. Their activity consists mainly of tissue building; no destructive process has been discovered. The protoplasm of plants is taken from the older, dying parts and is used again in tissue building and growth; the tissue does not decompose, and there is no waste product, as in flesh foods.

Dairy Products

Milk and milk products in the form of cheese, buttermilk, and yogurt contain the essential amino acids that make them complete protein. Cheese has the largest amount of available protein. Milk, buttermilk, and yogurt contain an average of 4–5 percent protein, and while their protein content is considerably lower than the other animal proteins, the usual serving is larger than the usual serving of more concentrated forms, and more of the protein is directly usable than in cheese.

Milk has always been criticized as being food for the nourishment of newborn mammals, not intended or fit for consumption after the period of nursing, which varies from one month to about one year.

It may be true that milk and milk products are an unnatural source of food, but their nutrient composition, digestibility, and amount of usable protein exceeds those of most other protein foods. Many adults, however, have exhausted their ability to digest milk—lacking rennin in the digestive juices—and develop inflammation of the mucous membranes in the nose and throat, constipation, and gas. Buttermilk and yogurt are usually easier to digest, because they have soured, they contain less milk sugar (lactose).

Cheese, in its many varieties, is the product of curdled milk, more or less skimmed. It comes fresh or cooked; may also be fermented, salted, or unsalted; and contains varying amounts of fat determined by the quality of the milk from which it is made. Fresh nonfermented cheeses are made from cows' milk that is usually pasteurized and salted. Many of the European cheeses are manufactured from goat and sheep milk and are generally considered better quality protein. All cheeses are concentrated foods, rich in protein, fat, and salt. Cheese requires an average of 3½ hours to digest, is highly acid-forming, and constipates. It takes about seven ounces of concentrated cheese to provide two ounces of usable protein. Seven ounces of concentrated cheese also supplies more than 1,000 calories, half of which come from the fat, and more salt than your body can handle and causes severe, damaging constipation. Because of the fat, salt, and abundant calories, cheese should be eaten in moderation and combined with green leafy vegetables or acid fruit.

Fresh cottage cheese made from whole raw milk, unsalted, is the most wholesome cheese. It contains about 20 percent protein and is low in fat and calories. Ten ounces of cottage cheese will supply two ounces of usable protein. It is superior in nutritive value, with regard to supplying protein, vitamins and minerals, to the best cuts of meat and is free from animal waste matter. It takes three hours to be digested.

Milk and dairy products that are raw and unpasteurized have

nutrient value higher than pasteurized products, because they have not been boiled away, and do not form acid as do other proteins and all other dairy products.

Eggs

Eggs are the most usable form of protein, most closely resembling the protein makeup of the human body. They provide about 12 percent protein, but at the same time they provide more than 12 percent fat, and are highly acid-forming. There is 20 percent more protein in the yolks, and the yolks contain all the fat. Muscle builders and athletes who depend on muscle endurance refuse all dairy products because they feel that milk products marble the muscles with useless fat. However, they will eat the whites of eggs for their high protein and low fat content, despite high acid.

It takes eight eggs (16 ounces) to make two ounces of usable protein. Digestion time is 2½ hours. Since cooled off egg whites are very hard to break down, hard-boiled eggs are more difficult to digest, so soft-boiling is the preferred cooking method to facilitate the digestion and the utilization of protein.

Most authorities recommend that eggs be eaten no more than two or three times a week. Eggs should be combined with green leafy vegetables, which are strongly alkaline, to counteract high acid. The combination of eggs and bread is an especially damaging mix, due to the eggs being hard to digest and the starch readily forming gas, thus producing excessive acid formation. Beware of the consequences.

Vegetable Protein

Almost all vegetables have noticeable amounts of protein. They contain an average of 1–6 percent protein. Green leafy vegetables play an indispensable part in the nutrition of man because they furnish the necessary vitamins and alkaline elements. In all diets that consist largely of cereal, flesh, and dairy foods a liberal supply of green vegetables is absolutely necessary to prevent overacidity of the blood.

Vegetables may be divided into five classes of which the most common are:

Class 1: Fruit-Bearing Vegetables

Chayote	Peppers
Cucumbers	Pumpkins
Eggplant	Squash
Melons	Tomatoes
Okra	

Class 2: Green Vegetables

Artichokes	Kale
Beet Leaves	Kohlrabi
Broccoli	Lettuce
Brussels sprouts	Mustard leaves
Cabbage	Parsley
Cauliflower	Rhubarb
Celery	Sorrel
Chard	Spinach
Dandelions	Watercress
Endive	

Class 3: Succulent Roots and Bulbs

Asparagus	Kohlrabi
Beets	Leeks
Black salsify	Onions
Carrots	Parsnips
Celery root	Radishes
Chives	Rutabagas
Garlic	Salsify
Horseradish	Turnips

Class 4: Starch-bearing Roots and Tubers

Arrowroot	Potatoes
Cassava	Sweet Potatoes
Dasheen	Taro
Jerusalem artichokes	Yams

Class 5: Mushrooms, Fungi, Lichens, Algae (Seaweeds)

Fruit-bearing vegetables contain from 90 to 95 percent water, are low in calories, and are rich in the alkaline salts: potash, lime, magnesia, and iron. The tomato, like other acid vegetables and fruits, is potentially alkaline after being digested and oxidized in the body. If improperly digested, the fruit-bearing vegetables may cause toxic discomfort that can become quite uncomfortable. It is therefore advisable to eat the fruit-bearing vegetables alone or to combine them with green leafy vegetables. When combined with starch, the oxalic acid in the tomato will stop the secretion of the starch-splitting enzyme, ptyalin, and render the entire combination indigestible. Tomatoes combined with protein will inhibit the secretion of pepsin necessary for reducing the protein into amino acids.

Melons undergo no digestion in the stomach. The little digestion they require takes place in the intestines. If melons are combined with foods that are broken down in the stomach, they will ferment rapidly, producing gas and discomfort.

Green leafy vegetables contain only a small percentage of solid nourishment, but they are rich in alkaline salts—especially soda, lime, and iron—and are indispensable for maintaining the alkaline level of the blood. They should be eaten raw to make full use of their high vitamin and mineral content and to derive the most benefit from their fibrous structure in keeping the digestive system clean and working freely.

The alkaline salts enter the vegetables from the roots in the form of ions, or electrically charged molecules, and circulate through the plant fluids and tissues. Eating fresh, raw vegetables in the form of combination salads not only supplies nutrients but also provides alkaline salts that supply vital electricity in the form of negatively and positively charged ions called *electrolytes*. A constant osmotic pressure between the cells is maintained by these electrolytes, which is as important to the life of the cells as are proteins and vitamins.

When vegetables are fried the organic salts are no longer found in ionized form, and when vegetables are boiled they lose 5–10 percent of their protein and more than 50 percent of their alkaline salts. Therefore, vegetables should be steamed or baked if they are not eaten raw.

Young green vegetables provide the most protein. However, due to their average of 90 percent water content, such a large volume of green vegetables would have to be consumed to supply necessary protein that they must be viewed as a secondary source.

Succulent roots and bulbs, such as beets, onions and asparagus, are 75–90 percent water, 1–6 percent protein, and 10–15 percent starch. Although they are not as rich in the alkaline elements as the green vegetables, they contain a sufficient amount to make them valuable.

Starch-bearing roots and tubers are an average of 76 percent water, 2 percent protein, and 21 percent starch. The potato, sweet potato, and yam make up the most important part of this vegetable group. The potato is a staple food for millions of people throughout the world, and next to cereals is probably the most important food product of the world.

The percentage of iron and lime in potatoes is small, and they should therefore be eaten in combination with green leafy vegetables to make up for the deficiency. More than 20 percent of the nutrient is discarded when the skin is removed for cooking, and boiling the remaining part removes another 50–60 percent. The best way to cook white potatoes, sweet potatoes, and yams is to bake them slowly, being sure to eat the white potato with the skin. There is little fiber in potatoes, and eating the skin adds fiber. For the most part, however, potatoes and other starch-bearing foods should be considered constipating, which is another reason to combine them with raw vegetable salads. Potatoes are alkaline-forming.

Nut Protein

From three to four ounces of nuts, well chewed or in the form of unroasted nut butter, will supply all the protein the average adult requires in one day. moreover, the protein of nuts is of greater biological value for the renewal of body tissue than the protein from the muscular tissues of a dead animal, with all of its waste problems.

Unroasted nuts and nut butter also contain a high percentage of fat combined with alkaline salts in the purest form, and for this reason they are superior to the extracted or isolated animal and/or vegetable fats. A certain amount of fat is necessary to regulate the body heat, to keep the arteries flexible, to keep the bowels regular, to carry valuable fat-soluble vitamins, and to protect and hold the vital organs in place.

All fats slow down digestion and combine poorly with proteins because they lower the amount of pepsin and hydrochloric acid in the digestive juices by as much as 50 percent. The natural combination of high protein and high fat in nuts and seeds, along with a high percentage of fiber, makes nuts difficult to digest. They must be chewed very well, eaten in small quantities, and combined only with vegetables, fruit, or cheese. The digestibility of nuts is increased as much as 10 percent when eaten in the form of nut butter.

The pecan contains the largest amount of fat, about 70 percent, followed closely by the hickory nut, Brazil nut, filbert, and pine nut, which contain more than 60 percent fat. The pignolia ranks the highest in the amount of protein, containing nearly 34 percent; the peanut is next, with 28 percent; the butternut, almond, and pistachio all contain over 20 percent protein, which surpasses the best cuts of meat.

All nuts, with the exception of Brazil nuts, filberts, and black walnuts, are alkaline-forming. Do not combine them with other protein or with starch. Their time for digestion ranges from 2½ to 3½ hours. Care should be taken when selecting nuts to avoid ones that have been sulphured in the process of their drying and roasting. Sulphuring is a method of speeding drying time by exposing the product to burning sulphur fumes. Sulphuring is used more extensively in processing dried fruits to keep them from looking dried out. Sulphuring of any food is extremely harmful. It adds sulphuric acid to the food, which is an additional highly poisonous nutrient killer in the body.

The table on page 39 shows the protein value of the most popular nuts.

All nuts are really seeds. The difference between nuts and seeds is slight, seeds generally having greater amounts of calcium, potassium, and iron. Both should be eaten in moderation, well

Nut	Protein Percentage	Calories Per 3½ Oz.	Acid/Alk.
Almond	18.6	598	ALK (strong)
Beechnut	19.4	568	alk
Black Walnut	20.5	628	alk
Brazil Nut	14.3	629	acid
Butternut	27.9	629	alk
Caraway Seeds	19.8	____	____
Cashew	17.2	561	alk
Chestnut	2.9	377	ALK (strong)
Coconut	3.5	346	alk
English Walnut	14.8	651	acid
Filbert	12.6	635	acid
Flax Seeds	22.6	____	____
Hemp Seeds	18.2	____	____
Hickory	13.2	673	alk
Macadamia	7.8	691	alk
Mustard Seeds	27.6	____	____
Peanut (actually a legume)	26.3	568	acid
Pecan	9.2	657	alk
Pignolia	33.9	552	alk
Pine Nut	13.0	635	alk
Pistachio	19.3	594	alk
Poppy Seeds	19.4	____	____
Pumpkin and Squash Seeds	29.0	553	alk
Sesame Seeds	18.6	582	alk
Sunflower Seeds	24.0	560	alk

chewed. Keep in mind that nuts and seeds are high in calories and can be consumed in great quantity if treated as a snack food.

Legume Protein

Legumes include soybeans, dried peas, dried beans, and lentils. They have a high percentage of protein, ranging from 18 to 35 percent, with the soybean heading the list, which also contains 16–18 percent fat. Because of their high protein and carbohydrate (starch) content and low amount of alkaline elements, legumes are highly acid-forming and should be eaten moderately and always combined with raw vegetable salads to add as much alkaline element as possible.

Legumes are difficult to digest, even when prepared properly, diminishing their potential as usable protein. The difficulty is that the nutrients are enclosed in cellulose cells (woody fiber), which interfere with absorption and makes them likely to ferment in the intestines. This rapid fermentation and tough cellulose irritate the intestine, which produces gas and increases peristaltic movement. If a large quantity is eaten, movement through the bowel is rapid, which produces flatulence and diarrhea, thereby decreasing absorption of nutrients and water.

The proper preparation of legumes is of great importance to assure their digestion and assimilation. They should be soaked in soft water overnight, brought to a boil in the same water, (to retain as many vitamins and minerals as possible), covered, and simmered for a minimum of two hours. Cooking beans under pressure is a preferred method, since it is faster and loses fewer nutrients. Digestion time for prepared legumes ranges from 2½ to 3½ hours.

The table on page 41 shows the protein, starch (carbohydrate), and calorie values of the most popular legumes.

Although legumes have large amounts of protein, they are not complete proteins. They score low on more than one essential amino acid, which reduces their usable protein by 50 percent. Add to this their basic indigestibility and high calories, and they become only a fair source of protein.

The soybean seems to be the most important legume, with a higher percentage of usable protein and a higher amino acid content than other beans. It has been used to develop a product called *tofu*. Tofu is a concentrated soybean curd with the crude fiber and water-soluble carbohydrates (starch) removed. Tofu is digested easily, is low in calories and saturated fats, and is 50 percent higher in calcium than milk. The protein in tofu has a complete complement of amino acids and resembles the protein found in chicken. An eight-ounce serving of tofu supplies more

Bean	Protein Percentage	Starch Percentage	Calories Per 3½ Oz.	Acid/Alk.
Broadbean, dried	25.1	58.2	338	alk
Broadbean, fresh	8.4	17.8	105	alk
Cowpea, dried	22.8	61.7	343	alk
Cowpea, fresh	9.0	21.8	127	alk
Garbanzo, dried	20.5	61.0	360	alk
Lentil, dried	24.7	60.1	340	ACID (strong)
Lima, dried	20.4	64.0	345	ALK (strong)
Lima, fresh	8.4	22.1	123	alk
Mung, dried	24.2	60.3	340	alk
Mung, sprouts	3.8	6.6	35	alk
Pea, dry	24.1	60.3	340	alk
Pea, fresh	6.3	14.4	884	alk
Peanut	26.0	17.6	568	ACID (strong)
Pinto, dried	22.9	63.7	349	alk
Red, dried	22.5	61.9	343	alk
Snap	1.9	7.1	32	alk
Soybean, dried	34.1	33.5	403	alk
Soybean, fresh	10.9	13.2	134	alk
Soybean, sprouts	6.2	5.3	46	ALK (strong)
White, dried	22.3	61.3	340	acid

than 11 grams of usable protein at a far lower cost than any other protein source.

Meat, fish, and poultry contain 20 times more pesticide residual than legumes, and dairy products contain more than four times the residual.

Cereal Protein (Grains)

Cereals are the dry seeds of matured plants in which nature has stored the elements for the germination and growth of the embryo plant until the roots, stems, and leaves grow strong enough to absorb nourishment directly from the soil and air. For this purpose the seeds carry a large percentage of protein, carbohydrates (starch), gluten, fat, organic salts, and vitamins.

Cereals supply almost half the protein in the world, though many authorities consider them less than the best food for man. They are acid-forming, incomplete proteins, and high in calories. Although grains are not as acid-forming as meat, fish, and eggs, they nevertheless increase the acidity of the blood and therefore should be combined with green leafy vegetables.

The major cereals, in their order of popularity are: rice, corn, wheat, oats, barley, rye, buckwheat, millet, and sorghum. Triticale is a newly developed cross between rye and wheat and is reported to have 17 percent protein. Wheat, rye, and oats contain the most protein of all grains, ranging from 9 to 14 percent; wild rice has 14 percent, and white rice 7 percent.

The following list shows the protein, starch (carb), and calorie values of the leading cereals.

Grain	Percentage Protein	Percentage Starch	Calories per 3½ Oz.
Barley	9.6	77.6	348
Durum	12.7	70.1	332
Millet	9.9	72.9	327
Oatmeal/Rolled Oats, cooked	2.0	9.7	55.
Rice, cooked	2.5	25.5	119
Rye	19.4	77.9	359
White enriched flour	10.5	76.1	364
Whole-wheat flour	13.3	71.0	333

weak

Because grains are ~~week~~ in some of the essential amino acids, the usable protein is reduced by as much as 50 percent. The one exception is rice. The available, usable protein in rice is as high as in beef. Wheat germ and rice germ are high in usable protein, and oatmeal and buckwheat provide a good amount. Pastas and breads supply little protein and cannot be considered a source.

Generally grains are difficult to digest because of their strong combination of starch and protein. Eating too much cereal product will cause digestive disturbance, high acid levels in the blood, and a desire to eat more. The time for digestion of grains ranges from two hours for rice to four hours for wheat.

PROPER COMBINING—PROTEINS

The purpose of this book is to explore the process of developing superior health by selecting and combining foods that provide necessary nutrients aith the least amount of toxic residue. This will lighten the load on the digestive system, improve elimination, and maintain a high alkaline level in the blood.

It is from protein sources that most toxic substances are derived. Proteins, for the most part, are acid-forming, and these acid-forming elements have to be minimized by overwhelming them with acid-binding alkaline foods. Protein is the most essential nutrient for living, but at the same time it is the most poisonous. Special care must be taken when selecting protein sources, determining amounts, and combining protein with other foods.

The character of the digestive juice secreted corresponds with the character of the food to be digested, and each food calls for its own specific modification of the digestive juice.

It follows that complex mixtures of foods will necessarily impair the efficiency of digestion. This is especially true with protein foods because of their highly complex nature and their need for precisely timed stages of digestion.

As noted earlier, pepsin is the enzyme that initiates the digestion of all proteins. Pepsin acts in an acid environment, beginning in the stomach, and is weakened or destroyed by alkaline elements, cold temperature, fat, or too much acid.

For digestive efficiency and the best nutrient absorption, protein food is best eaten alone, combined with no other food. In combination, it is wise to combine protein foods with green leafy vegetable salads and/or nonstarchy vegetables to offset the acid production and to add fiber for healthy and rapid elimination.

Eat Protein and Starch at Separate Meals

This is the first rule in proper food combining. As discussed earlier, the acid environment necessary for pepsin to work on protein is established by the outpouring of hydrochloric acid in the stomach. Starch digestion begins in the mouth with the secretion of ptyalin in the saliva. But hydrochloric acid in the stomach destroys any ptyalin mixed with starch when it is swallowed, completely halting the digestion of that starch in the stomach. Then the undigested starch in the stomach absorbs pepsin and either stops or retards the digestion of protein. There is resulting fermentation of the starch, significant reduction of available amino acids from the protein, and absorption of chemical toxins into the blood. The putrefied, compacted refuse then paralyzes the movement of the bowels, retaining waste, which causes constipation and lays the foundation for toxemia, enervation, and disease.

It has been suggested that the stomach can handle a small amount of food with the natural combination of protein and starch by mixing the food with the gastric juices in the lower end of the stomach and separating the starch in the upper end, still under the influence of the saliva. The stomach does this with difficulty, however, as illustrated by the difficulty experienced in digesting natural protein-starch combinations such as beans, grains, and nuts. If the stomach does have this capability, starch may be eaten at the same time with protein if the protein is eaten first and allowed to digest in the lower end of the stomach and the starch eaten separately and last, stopping at the upper end of the stomach. Small amounts of protein and starch would have to be eaten to accommodate this separating function so as not to force the stomach to combine the food at both ends from volume alone. Even under ideal conditions, the combination of protein and starch makes digestion difficult. The separating ability of the stomach may be kept in mind for those times when you purposely deviate from the properly combined meal or when you are caught in an eating situation in which you have no control over the food and you want to minimize the damage.   *DO THIS*

Eating protein and starch at separate meals eliminates combinations like eggs and toast, meat and cheese sandwiches, and drinking milk with starch meals.

do not do. this

Eat Protein and Acids at Separate Meals

Lemon juice, vinegar, tomatoes, and other acids added to salads and eaten with a protein meal or used in the preparation of protein limit the secretion of hydrochloric acid, weaken the power of the protein enzyme pepsin, and result in poor protein digestion.

Animal protein—flesh, dairy, egg—is so complex and unstable that any interference with its digestion causes rapid putrefaction in the warm bacterial environment of the stomach, and putrefying animal food produces the most virulent toxins.

The exception to this rule is the combination of nuts, avocados, or cheese with acid fruits. Nuts and cheeses contain a high content of fat or oil, do not decompose as rapidly as other protein food, and are not delayed by the presence of acids because they remain in the stomach longer to begin with.

Eat Proteins and Fats at Separate Meals

The presence of fat—butter, cream, margarine, vegetable oils, bacon, bacon grease, lard, etc.—in the stomach inhibits the secretion of gastric juice, lowering the amounts of hydrochloric acid and pepsin in the gastric juice, and retards protein digestion for two hours or more.

The presence of fat in fat meats (such as lamb, steak or prepared meats), fried meats or fish, fried eggs, milk, nuts, cheese, and other fat foods is the reason that these foods take longer to digest than foods with little fat content.

If fat must be combined with protein, or if a high-fat protein is eaten, raw green vegetable salads will help counteract the inhibiting effect of the fat. Uncooked cabbage is particularly effective in helping to digest fat.

Protein foods containing significant amounts of fat are, in order of amount, bacon, most nuts, cheese, cream, pork, ham, beef, lamb chops, and turkey.

Eat Proteins and Sugars at Separate Meals

Sugars—commercial sugar, raw sugar, honey, fruit, fruit sugar, molasses, date sugar—inhibit both gastric secretion and the movement of the stomach needed for mixing and churning the food with the digestive juices. When combined with protein food, sugar limits the secretion of hydrochloric acid and pepsin and assures an incomplete mix of the little digestive juice that is present with the protein, resulting in poor digestion.

Sugars undergo no digestion in the mouth or in the stomach. They are digested in the intestine. When sugars are eaten alone they are not held in the stomach for long. But when they are combined with protein (or starch) they are held up in the stomach, slow the process of digestion, and begin to ferment, to pollute the environment, and to destroy the protein. Fruit, while it is a most nutritious, cleansing food, behaves like any sugar in the digestive process, and with few exceptions should not be combined with protein or starch. A fruit dessert following a protein meal will cause gas and discomfort; following a meal including potatoes or bread, fruit will rapidly ferment with the starch and possibly disable digestion for the next two days. Fruit pies will almost always cause indigestion.

Experiments have shown that finishing a meal with cream and sugar in a drink will delay the digestion of the meal for more than three hours.

Eat Only One Concentrated Protein Food at a Meal

The chemical makeup and digestive disintegration of proteins are the most complex of all foods. The significant feature of protein digestion is the stages of disintegration that protein foods must go through to break out the necessary amino acids. These stages are disrupted easily, and they lose their effectiveness when proteins are combined with foods that have conflicting digestive requirements. The process is confused just as easily by combining unlike proteins.

For example, the strongest enzyme is secreted for flesh protein during the first hour of digestion and poured out on milk in the last hour of digestion. Eggs receive the strongest secretion at a different time; cheese has still another cycle; nuts have different timing.

Overcrowding nutrition will have the same effect of disabling digestion as miscombinations.

Combining like proteins—flesh with flesh, nuts with nuts, cheese with cheese—shouldn't present any problem, but digestion will be slowed and distress may result when combining unlike proteins such as:

DO NOT DO THIS

- Flesh with eggs
- Flesh with cheese
- Flesh with nuts
- Eggs with milk
- Eggs with nuts
- Eggs with cheese
- Cheese with nuts
- Milk with anything

Milk, while it is a complete source of highly usable protein, has traditionally caused digestive problems for many people. Many researchers are adamantly against using milk in any form after being weaned from mother's milk. Their argument is sound and is based on the body's inability to manufacture rennin, the pancreatic enzyme necessary to digest milk, after the first year or two of life. Upon entering the stomach milk coagulates, forming curds that surround the particles of other food present and insulate them from the working of digestion until the curds are digested. Nature didn't provide for man to be supplied with milk beyond childhood. Without question, milk is mucous-forming. Many adults experience gas, diarrhea, or constipation, nausea, and acidosis from drinking only a few ounces of milk.

As you develop a feel for proper food combining you will lose your taste for highly toxic foods like meat, cheese, and sugar. While milk may not be the best food for you, raw milk, raw milk products (raw cottage cheese), and soured dairy products (buttermilk, yogurt, kefir) are easier to digest, are alkaline-forming, and are a valuable source of protein.

An additional disadvantage of combining more than one protein at the same meal is the distinct tendency to overeat concentrated foods. All concentrated foods, such as meat, fish, fowl, eggs, bread, pasta and potatoes, have a stimulating effect on the body, and this stimulation can easily become addicting, can overcrowd nutrition, and can lead to obesity. Overweight people are addicted to concentrated foods. The reason they are unsuccessful at controlling weight is because they are unsuccessful at controlling that addiction. Eating only one concentrated protein at any meal will minimize the opportunity to overeat and to build addictive patterns.

CONCLUSIONS ABOUT PROTEIN

How Much Is Needed

While proteins in their different forms are essential in maintaining health, the required amount for one's daily need is subject to continuing controversy.

Singular muscular tissues consist mainly of protein, and muscles make up most of the body, early students of nutrition assumed that protein from food was the source of muscular energy. This idea has been proved wrong, yet some nutritionists still advise eating more protein than is necessary for the repair and building of tissue as a safety measure in case reserves become depleted.

Nitrogen is the working component of protein, and nitrogen cannot be stored up in the body to any great extent. Too much nitrogen in the blood acts as a poison that overtaxes the liver and kidneys trying to eliminate it and may very well be the cause of emotional disorder, fibroid tumors, hardening of the arteries, infection, and quite possibly cancer.

The oxidation (burning) of food elements usually takes place in the active tissues (muscles), but it does not seem to occur at the expense of the protein in the living cells. Only the carbon contained in protein is used in the production of heat and energy, while the system has to excrete the surplus of nitrogen. The breaking up of the highly complicated protein molecule and the elimination of the nitrogenous end products taxes vitality.

The fuel value of protein, which contains 50 to 55 percent carbon, is not greater than that of an equal amount of sugar or starch. Heat and energy are supplied most efficiently from complex carbohydrates in the form of fruits and vegetables.

Alkaline elements in the blood protect the protein in the tissues against premature disintegration. Weight can be maintained and health and endurance increased on an alkaline diet furnishing even less than two ounces of protein per day. The mammary glands of the human mother supply less protein as an infant grows older. After six months the percentage of protein in mother's milk decreases from 2 percent to just 1 percent.

The exact amount of protein necessary for any one person cannot be determined exactly. It is certain, however, that more efficient digestion will permit the absorption of more nutrients. Proper food combining will immediately improve the efficiency of the digestive process, breaking out more amino acids from less protein, resulting in less nitrogenous waste to pollute the blood and to overtax the organs.

The figures published by government research organizations recommending minimum protein requirements are determined by the amount of nitrogen found in the urine and feces of test individuals who have been denied protein food. The amount of nitrogen loss is projected to be the amount of protein food any particular person of that weight needs to replace body protein lost through degeneration. This projection of the minimum protein requirement is then recommended in grams of protein needed each day for the maintenence of the body.

The measurement doesn't take into account the body's utilization of protein, health, stress, temperature, age, and other factors. The efficiency of body function can be the only determinant of the need for restoration, and at this point that is not measurable.

After food combining for a while you will be able to determine your own need for protein and will develop an instinct for the best sources. The condition of your hair, nails, and skin is a good indication of the adequacy of your protein. Unfortunately, these areas are the last to show deficiency or improvement. The ease in which a cut or an abrasion heals would be a better indication of whether you are getting enough protein. Just a general body awareness and self-communication will tell you everything you need to know. Food combining will open that communication.

ABOUT CALORIES IN PROTEIN

Most people know whether a food is high in calories or low in calories. With few exceptions, just looking at the density of a food can tell you about its caloric content. To make a study of the caloric content of a certain number of ounces of the various foods is a waste of time. It is far more productive to think about alkaline elements in food than to think about the calories. It will serve you better to know how long it takes to digest a certain food than to know how many calories that food contains.

It is equally meaningless to study the calorie charts to determine how many calories a person with your bone structure can consume each day without gaining weight. It is an exercise in futility to try to measure your caloric intake without checking into a hospital where all your food and liquid is premeasured in grams and served in plastic packages.

It is enough to know that your body needs at least 1,000 calories a day to maintain a high energy level. The exact amount is unimportant; your body will let you know if you need more or less.

Every gram of protein available in a food costs four calories. Every gram of carbohydrate also costs four calories. Each gram of fat costs nine calories. When you are selecting food just for the protein value, the highest amount of usable protein provided with the least amount of carbohydrates and fats will cost the fewest calories. This, of course, isn't the way protein should be selected all the time because of our need for carbohydrate and fat, but the concept will give you a way to work with this calorie cost accounting method.

Protein Food	Calories/ Usable Gram of Protein	Protein Food	Calories/ Usable Gram of Protein
Chicken	7	Legumes/Tofu	15
Dairy/Cottage Cheese	10	Nuts/Cashews	55
Dairy/Egg	14	Nuts/Peanuts	49
Flour/Rye	34	Seafood/Haddock	5
Flour/Wheat	41	Seafood/Swordfish	8
Grain/Brown rice	69	Steak	14
Grain/Oatmeal	41	Veg/Potato	60
Legumes/Garbanzos	40	Veg/Spinach	18

Whatever your maximum allowance for calories is, proper food combining will increase it. If your food processing and elimination systems work efficiently, you won't store fat. You will eat less food and will benefit more from the food that you eat.

Ideally, your diet should consist of 75 percent raw fruit and vegetables and 25 percent concentrated foods in the form of starch, fat, and protein. Even if you do not achieve this, the ratio will relieve you of having to think about calories.

COMPARING THE COST OF PROTEIN FOODS

The best dollar investment in usable protein is dairy products. Within this group dried nonfat milk solids are by far the least expensive, followed by cottage cheese, eggs, buttermilk, and whole milk. Cheese, which appears to be expensive, is actually relatively inexpensive when considering investing in usable protein, and yogurt, while appearing inexpensive, is almost as costly as meat.

Dried beans, peas, and lentils remain a low-cost source of protein despite the fact that they offer little usable protein because of a low contribution of some of the essential amino acids. Larger amounts have to be eaten to achieve the body's requirement for protein.

Wheat, rye, and oat grains prove to be good investments in usable protein when purchased in bulk and made into bread and cereals at home.

Seafood is generally a good investment, and even the more expensive varieties like crab and crayfish prove to be relatively inexpensive when you consider the smaller amount necessary to supply large quantities of usable protein. Some seafood, in fact, supplies usable protein less expensively than beans.

Nuts and seeds have a wide range, with cashews costing as much as beef and lamb, and peanuts and peanut butter costing as little as wheat flour and milk for the supply of usable protein. Raw nuts and seeds are superior in nutritional value to roasted and salted products and are considerably less expensive.

Chicken is the least expensive in the flesh food group, followed by pork, beef, lamb, and veal.

5

Starch Combinations

WHAT STARCH IS

Starch is just one form of carbohydrate and is of no use to the human body until it is digested and turned into blood sugar to fuel the brain and nervous system and to provide energy for the muscles and heat for the organs of the body.

Although the body has a specific need for carbohydrates, there is no specific need for starch. It is rather difficult to digest, it ferments easily, and it is decidedly habit-forming. When cooked properly, however, starchy vegetables can provide valuable nutrients and even protein.

THE NEED FOR CARBOHYDRATES

The body needs carbohydrates from sugars, starches, and vegetables to produce energy, to keep the body temperature sufficiently high, and to allow the protein replacement in the cells to proceed uninterrupted.

If the body is not supplied with enough carbohydrates to meet its energy requirements, protein will be diverted from its primary function of rebuilding tissue and will be wasted as cheap energy fuel. Burning protein for energy is inefficient. Protein doesn't make good energy fuel, and when it is forced to do that task it produces waste that overtaxes liver and kidneys and acidifies the blood.

Carbohydrates are absolutely necessary to achieve superior health. As much as 75 percent of the diet should be carbohydrate vegetable foods. Starch is just one form of carbohydrate—a concentrated form that should be prepared with care in order to retain the nutrients and should be eaten in small quantities but not every day.

METABOLIZING STARCH

Because starch digestion begins in the mouth, as explained earlier, thoroughly chewing and mixing saliva with the starch is extremely important. Starch is difficult to digest and requires time to be completely saturated with saliva. Ptyalin begins breaking the starch down into maltose, which is further acted on in the intestine by maltase and then converted into simple sugar dextrose and further into glucose. Again, the action of ptyalin upon starch is preparatory, because maltase cannot act on starch in its original form. Starch that escapes this preparatory breakdown into maltose gets one more opportunity to be acted on after it leaves the stomach to journey through the intestine, by the pancreatic enzyme amylase.

UNDIGESTED STARCH

This normal process of digestive events can be halted from the very beginning if ptyalin does not contact the starch. Undigested starch thus delayed in the stomach will begin to ferment quickly and will become gaseous. Then it will pass into the intestines, where the emitting poisons will be absorbed by the blood, contributing acids to a system that needs to be alkaline.

In addition to producing toxic gases that are paralyzing to the digestive system and poisonous to the body, undigested starch absorbs fluids in both the stomach and the intestines. In the stomach undigested starch will tend to absorb other digestive juices and limit the potential of other foods for being processed properly. In the intestines undigested starch will absorb water and cause constipation.

Starchy foods are predominantly acid-forming. To offset this potential for acid formation, green leafy vegetables should be combined with starch in a ratio of four to one.

DIFFERENCES IN STARCH FOODS

Starches are classified as grains, legumes, and roots and tubers (potatoes).

The principal grains are wheat, corn, oats, barley, rye, and rice. No grains, even in their natural state, contain enough alkaline to prevent an increase of acidity in the blood.

Starch-bearing vegetables include potatoes, yams, sweet potatoes, hubbard squash, banana squash, pumpkins, artichokes, chestnuts, caladium root, and arrowroot. Cauliflower, beets, carrots, rutabaga, and salsify are vegetables with a moderate amount of starch. All starch-bearing vegetables are alkaline-forming.

Legumes—dried beans and peas, peanuts, and lentils—are all alkaline-based in their raw state but become acid-formers when cooked.

All starch foods are rich in carbohydrates and have the same four calories per gram as protein but are difficult to digest. The following review of starch foods will provide a working knowledge of what each has to offer when combined properly.

Grains

Whole grains are made up of three different parts. The germ is the heart of the grain and is the part that sprouts when the seed is planted. It is rich in B and E vitamins, protein, carbohydrates, unsaturated fat, and minerals, especially iron. The endosperm makes up the largest part of the grain. It is composed chiefly of carbohydrates in the form of starch, with some low-quality protein and traces of vitamins and minerals. The bran is the covering of the grain. It is composed of cellulose, a carbohydrate roughage found in all plants, along with traces of B vitamins, iron, and protein.

While the whole grain is edible, the bran and germ are often removed during milling to reduce the chance of rancidity and to extend storage time. With the removal of the germ and bran, as much as 75 percent of all vitamins and minerals are lost. Refined flours milled in this way are required to be enriched in order to qualify as a food. Thiamine, riboflavin, and iron are added during processing.

Wheat

Winter wheat has less gluten (protein) and more starch than spring wheat. It is softer and preferred by the manufacturers of pasta and semolina. The mineral matter of both varieties is almost entirely composed of phosphate of potash and phosphate of magnesium with small proportions of soda, chlorine, and lime.

Whole-grain flour is the product of the first milling of the whole grain and contains the germ of the grain and most of the nutrients. Whole-grain flour must be refrigerated to prevent rancidity. However, whole-grain breads should be stored at room temperature or frozen until used because refrigerated bread loses moisture and quickly becomes stale.

All-purpose flour is a blend of different wheat grains. Bleached flour has been whitened for the purpose of making more uniform and attractive bakery products, but it cannot support life, as bleaching destroys everything necessary for good nutrition.

There are 333 calories in 3½ ounces of whole-wheat flour, which is 71 percent starch, 8 percent usable protein, and 2 percent unsaturated fat. The digestion time is 3¾ hours. Wheat is highly acid-forming.

Rye

Rye contains less gluten than wheat but is richer in silicone and flourine, which are important in the formation of the enamel of the teeth. Rye flour is noted for its distinctive taste and is often combined with wheat flour to make a tastier bread.

There are 357 calories in 3½ ounces of rye flour, which contains 78 percent carbohydrates, including starch, 5 percent usable protein, and 1½ percent unsaturated fat. Digestion time is 3½ hours. Rye is more acid-forming than wheat.

Oats

Oats are the richest of all the grains in fat and in organic salts. Steel-cut oatmeal and flaked oats are the principal manufactured products. Oats have a gluten content similar to rye. While oats have 9 percent usable protein, they are usually eaten in a rolled form of cereal that is much lighter than whole grains and consequently provide much less nutrient by volume.

There are 55 calories in 3½ ounces of cooked oatmeal, which contains 10 percent carbohydrate, 1½ percent usable protein, and 1 percent fat. By comparison, there are 390 calories in 3½ ounces of uncooked rolled oats, which is 68 percent carbohydrate, 9 percent protein, and 7 percent fat. Oatmeal is acid-forming. Digestion time is 3½ hours.

Barley

Barley, like rye, has less gluten and is therefore not as well suited for making bread as is wheat. It is used extensively for stock feed and to make beer. Barley meal is used for porridge in the British Isles, and plain, hulled barley is often combined with other flours to make heavy bread.

Pot or Scotch barley has 348 calories in 3½ ounces and consists of 77 percent carbohydrates, 5 percent usable protein, and only 1 percent unsaturated fat. Digestion time is 3½ hours. Barley is acid-forming.

Corn

Corn is the leading cereal in the United States and in the Latin

American countries. It has less protein than wheat but is richer in fat, contained mostly in the germ.

Most of the cornmeal sold in the United States is degerminated and deprived of about 65 percent of its mineral matter. Corn flour, if made from the entire corn, is a wholesome food, and in combination with alkaline vegetables it makes a well-balanced meal.

Summer corn is most nutritious when it is young, before the maturing kernels store too much unsoluble starch, which is difficult to digest. Corn on the cob should be selected for its small white kernels. It begins turning to starch 24 hours after being picked.

Corn oil or maize oil is pressed from the germ of the corn and refined under high steam pressure and exposure to hydrogen, which is a deadly gas. This hydrogenated oil is heated to 400 degrees, destroying all important nutrients, for the sole purpose of protecting its shelf life and is suspected of contributing to high blood cholesterol and heart disease. Use only cold-pressed oil that is processed without heat or gases and always keep it refrigerated.

There are 96 calories in 3½ ounces of sweet corn, which is 22 percent carbohydrates, 2 percent usable protein, and 1 percent unsaturated fat. Digestion time is 3 hours. Corn is slightly alkaline.

Rice

The first milling of rice produces unpolished or brown rice, containing the germ and the outer layers of the kernel. As with other grains, the germ and the outer layers contain the vitamins and organic salts. When processed into white or polished rice, 75 percent of the nutrients are removed. Polished rice has been credited with causing the disease beriberi, due to its deficiency in B vitamins and minerals.

There are 119 calories in 3½ ounces of cooked brown rice, which is 77 percent carbohydrate, 3 percent usable protein, and less than 1 percent unsaturated fat. Digestion time is 2 hours. Rice is acid-forming.

Legumes

Legumes are plants that have edible seeds within a pod. They include peas, beans, lentils, and peanuts. Dried legumes are a source of iron, thiamine, riboflavin, niacin, and low-quality protein.

Because of their high content of protein and starch and their lack of alkaline elements, legumes become decidedly acid-forming when cooked. And because of their high cellulose fiber and their natural combination of protein and starch, legumes are difficult to digest. Dried legumes should be soaked overnight in soft or distilled water and then cooked in the same water to retain vitamins and minerals. Placing a cooked bean or pea on your tongue and mashing it against the roof of your mouth will tell you if it is sufficiently cooked. Soybeans should be soaked overnight in the refrigerator to prevent them from fermenting.

With the exception of soybeans, all dried legumes have an average of 140 calories in 3½ ounces when cooked and are 25 percent starch, 4 percent usable protein, and 2 percent unsaturated fat. Digestion time is 3 hours. Legumes are acid-forming and should be eaten with green leafy vegetable salads.

Soybeans have 130 calories per 3½ ounces cooked and are 10 percent starch, 7 percent usable protein, and 6 percent unsaturated fat. Digestion time for cooked soybeans is 3 hours.

The Potato

The potato is the most important starch-bearing vegetable. The white potato is high in potassium and vitamin C and should be baked without foil wrapping and eaten with the skin. When potatoes are peeled before cooking, about 20 percent of the nutrients are removed, and another 20 percent of the remaining nutrients are destroyed when they are boiled.

The potato has 93 calories in 3½ ounces and consists of 21 percent starch, 2 percent usable protein, and less than 1 percent fat. The digestion time is 2 hours. Potatoes are alkaline-forming.

Sweet Potato/Yam

The sweet potato and the yam have properties similar to the white potato, though they are not tubers. The carbohydrate content in the sweet potato and yam is higher due to a higher proportion of sugar with starch. Yams do not keep as well as white potatoes, but they are usually fresher from the soil when you buy them. They should be baked or steamed in their skins to retain nutrients.

The sweet potato and yam have approximately 140 calories in 3½ ounces and are 32 percent carbohydrate, 2 percent usable protein, and less than 1 percent fat. Digestion time is 3 hours. Sweet potatoes and yams are alkaline-forming.

The starch-bearing vegetables are easily digested but should be combined with raw green leafy vegetables to make up for their meager content of roughage.

PROPER COMBINING—STARCH

Starches provide the least amount of nutrients and wreak havoc with digestion when they are miscombined.

All starches are highly fermentable. They are so highly fermentable, in fact, that most distilled alcohol is made from grains and from potatoes. Just as in the making of alcohol, if starch sits in a warm, moist environment, it will begin to ferment, turn to alcohol, and emit gas immediately. Therefore, it is extremely important in food combining that starch foods be given careful attention. They must be combined with foods that will supplement their lack of roughage and must not be combined with foods that will delay their delicate and difficult digestion process.

If starch is not completely saturated with saliva containing ptyalin, thorough digestion will be sacrificed and fermentation will begin as soon as the food reaches the stomach. Ineffective chewing may well be a major reason for an intolerance to wheat and beans.

Eat Starch and Protein at Separate Meals

Saliva is 98 percent water. A mere 2 percent of saliva is the enzyme that makes this fluid alkaline—a delicate influence that can be destroyed easily.

Ptyalin, the starch-splitting enzyme, acts only in a milk alkaline environment to make starch ready for the final stage of digestion in the intestine. Two things can prevent ptyalin from performing its critical role of breaking down starch. One is to have the starch food pass through the mouth too quickly, and the other sure way is to change the oral environment from alkaline to acid.

Protein digestion requires the enzyme pepsin. Pepsin acts only in an acid environment and is destroyed in an alkaline environment. Combining starch with protein will stop starch digestion and will severely impair the digestion of the protein.

Foods that have a natural combination of protein and starch are the most difficult foods to digest. Poor digestion and allergic reactions caused by cereals, beans, and breads are common. The digestive system can process natural combinations of protein and starch with much difficulty, but when two foods are eaten with different and opposite digestive needs the adjustment process is overwhelmed and good digestion stops.

Do not combine any of the following foods.

- Bread with eggs
- Bread with meat, fish, chicken, cheese
- Potatoes with meat, fish, chicken, cheese
- Flour gravies with meat, fish, chicken
- Pasta with meat sauce, cheese, protein
- Beans with meat, chicken, or their stock
- Flour products with milk products

DO NOT DO THIS

This is the tough part. It means that poached eggs on toast is out, also chicken salad, turkey, grilled cheese, and hamburger sandwiches. Steak and a baked potato don't go together, nor do fish and chips, or melted cheese over potatoes or pasta. Leave the meat balls for another time and cover your spaghetti with marinara sauce, and leave off the grated cheese! The mixture of beans with meat in chili will cause trouble, and almost all of the Mexican dishes combining beans and tortillas with meat and cheese is sure to play havoc with even the heartiest digestive system.

Exceptions

There is a theory that starch and protein can be handled at the same time if the protein is eaten first and is allowed to go unmixed to the lower, or distal, end of the stomach, where the mixing with gastric juices takes place. Following this, the starch is able to be mixed with the saliva if it is eaten alone and passes to the quiescent, or upper, end of the stomach that is still under the influence of the saliva, where it can continue to digest without interference.

If this so-called segmenting of the stomach is possible, it can work only if a small volume of protein is followed by an equally small volume of starch so as not to mix the two together. Of course, the longer you wait between the two, the better. In any event, eating protein first and following it with starch is certainly better than mixing the two at the same time.

Eat Starches and Acids at Separate Meals

The mild alkalinity of saliva sets the stage for the secretion of ptyalin and the digestion of starch. With only 2 percent of the saliva providing this alkalinity, the slightest addition of any acid eaten along with starch will destroy the alkaline base and immediately stop the secretion of ptyalin.

For instance, there is enough acid in two teaspoons of vinegar to completely destroy the alkalinity of the saliva and prohibit any further secretion of ptyalin.

The acid of a raw tomato, lemon, lime, grapefruit, orange, berry, pineapple, or other sour fruit is sufficient to destroy ptyalin and to end the digestion of starch. Remember again that starch that enters the stomach without first being saturated with ptyalin will ferment quickly and will pollute the entire digestive tract, adding poisonous acids to the blood and paralyzing elimination.

Do not combine the following.

- Starch with acid fruit or acid fruit juice
- Starch with salads prepared with vinegar or acid fruit juice
- Starch with pickled vegetables

Exception

Cooked tomatoes or tomato sauce can be combined with starch (cooking tomatoes eliminates the acidity).

Eat Starch and Sugar at Separate Meals

Starch digestion begins in the mouth after the starch is saturated with saliva containing the enzyme ptyalin, and it continues under the influence of ptyalin in the stomach if conditions permit. Sugar—white sugar, brown sugar, maple syrup, cane sugar, honey, molasses, fructose, raw sugar, fruit, and fruit juice—requires no digestion in either the mouth or the stomach, yet it requires a heavy secretion of saliva that is devoid of ptyalin.

If starch is eaten with sugar of any kind, including fresh fruit, digestion of starch is stopped in two ways. First, the heavy flow of saliva stimulated by the sugar dilutes the ptyalin trying to reach the starch and renders it ineffective. Second, the sugar is delayed in the stomach to ferment while the starch uses the diluted saliva with weak enzymatic action to prepare it for the next stage of digestion in the intestine.

Combining sugar with starch thus ferments both of them. This is one of the miscombinations that is likely to cause immediate gastric discomfort.

Do not combine any of the following starches and sugars.

- Bread with jam, jelly, marmalade, honey
- Cereals with sugar
- Pancakes with syrup, sugar, honey
- Breads containing dried fruit
- Starch and sugar (cakes)
- Starch and sugar or fruit (pies and pastries)

DO NOT DO THIS

Fermentation caused by combining starch with sugar is inevitable. There is no way around those combinations that inhibit digestion and overtax the body with toxic waste. Maple sugar and honey offset fermentation somewhat with their traces of alkaline elements, so if temptation prevails, these would be the least harmful.

It will be a long time before your experience with food combining and your enthusiasm for perfect health will allow you to completely eliminate all the wonderful, sugary treats. You may never feel a need to eliminate them entirely. Sunday morning pancakes and maple syrup are a tradition in my house. Just understand that the body processes those combinations with difficulty, so either follow those exceptional meals with a raw vegetable salad or by skipping the following meal entirely.

Eat No More than One Starch at a Meal

Starches are highly concentrated acid-forming foods. The body overworks to digest them and to eliminate their toxic waste products. They also stimulate the nervous system the same way drugs do and are also addicting.

Starch addiction is not uncommon. Everyone knows someone who would prefer eating starch foods over any other kind of food. They are addicted to the stimulating effects of the toxins in starch and usually suffer from constipation, headaches, and low energy.

Limiting starch to only one at a meal will minimize the possibility of overeating it and developing an attachment to starchy foods that can only make controlling weight difficult and superior health more difficult to attain.

It is also a good practice to eat only one starch meal a day. The noon meal may prove best for having starch foods. Carbohydrates produce the energy necessary for thinking clearly and for feeling top-notch, so include them during the day when you need the most energy.

Drink Liquids before and Well after a Starch Meal

Drinking liquids with any meal dilutes digestive juices, which in turn slows digestion. Drinking liquids with a starch meal dilutes the ptyalin in the saliva and carries the enzyme away through the . stomach, leaving the starch undigested and fermentable.

It is best to drink no liquids 10–15 minutes before a starch meal and not again until two hours after.

Drinking cold or iced drinks within three hours after a meal of any kind will stop digestion until the temperature of the stomach returns to 100° F. Indigestion is sure to follow.

important

Limit Fats and Starches

The most commonly used fats are butter, cream, lard, vegetable oils, and bacon. Any food having starch as a base is less easily digested if mixed, cooked, or served with fat. When combined with fat, starch granules are less easily influenced by the ptyalin in saliva. However, fat is emulsified in the intestine, where the final stages of starch digestion take place, with both the fat and the starch under the influence of pancreatic enzymes. It may therefore be safe to assume that combining fats with starches will not disturb the digestion of either to any great extent except when the fat also contains a large amount of protein, like peanut butter and cream cheese.

Combine any of the following starches and fats:

- Bread with butter
- Potatoes with butter
- Potatoes with sour cream
- Bread with avocado
- Potatoes with bacon
- Bread with bacon

DO THIS

Do not combine these starches and fats:

- Bread with mayonnaise
- Bread with cream cheese
- Potatoes with mayonnaise
- Bread with peanut butter
- Starch with nuts

DO NOT DO THIS

CONCLUSIONS ABOUT STARCH

Starchy foods are the least important source of vitamins, minerals, and protein and are the most important source of trouble for the digestive system.

Starch overstimulates and taxes digestion even if eaten in moderation and combined with foods that do not interfere with its delicate processing. Overeating starch is a temptation because it excites the nervous system. Starch, like sugar, can become addicting. The body learns to crave stimulants if they are supplied regularly and will slowly but surely deteriorate from borrowed energy.

Overeating starch will tax digestion and can result in toxic poisoning that may lead to constipation, headaches, liver and heart disease, stomach and bowel disorders, gas distention, shortness of breath, coughing, piles, and bladder irritation accompanied by frequent urination.

These diseases of enervation can be avoided, and starchy foods may be enjoyed if they are eaten only two or three times a week, combined with raw vegetable salads that supply the alkaline elements missing in most starchy foods. Raw vegetable salads prevent fermentation and assure good elimination.

This warning about starch cannot be overemphasized. If it is combined with protein, sugar, or acids, it will cause trouble. That trouble is common to most people—fullness, gas, distention, sluggishness, constipation—and unfortunately is usually forgotten the next day. The real trouble is the resulting toxemia in the blood and tissues and the eventual enervation of vital nerve energy that erodes health and limits potential.

6

Applied Combinations

FORMING THE HABIT

Food combining will make a huge contribution to your health if it is learned well enough to become a habit and then practiced long enough to become automatic. If you approach the practice of food combining in the right way, you will be able to depend on yourself to make proper food choices without spending excessive time in planning, worrying, and feeling deprived.

There are no foods that you cannot eat while food combining. You may eat anything that you want, just as long as you remember two rules:

1. Foods, in combination, must be digestible.
2. Food must be in alkaline/acid balance.

By applying those two rules to everything you eat, you will develop the habit of properly combining food. Change is difficult. We feel comfortable with old behavior patterns, even though they

67

may be obsolete or even harmful. To make change permanent, steps must be taken to force the repetition of new behavior. Knowing theory or good reasons for change does not make change happen. Food combining is very logical, but to make it a part of your life it is necessary to modify your behavior.

REWARD AND PUNISHMENT

Behaviorists agree that most behavior is shaped by a system of reward and punishment. Every pattern anyone has ever learned was learned because there was always a prize for learning and a punishment for failure. Baseball players learn the intricate timing of hitting a baseball by being rewarded with cheering and with running to first base when they connect, and with booing and rejection when they strike out. Every form of behavior is shaped this way. Even the health enthusiast keeps running or exercising and attending to his sleep and diet because of the rewards of feeling good for all that discipline and the punishment of feeling slow, fat, and guilty if it is neglected too long.

Food combining will become automatic quickly and easily because inherent in its practice is a natural system of reward and punishment. All you have to do is let it work. Each time you eat anything, alone or in combination with another food, understand how that category of food is digested. Then know whether the food you are about to eat is acid-forming or alkaline-forming. That is all you need to do to kick off the natural reward and punishment system that comes with food combining. At the end of a meal the combinations that are acceptable to the digestive system will reward you with a pleasant sense of fullness, contentment, and a good feeling of knowing that you are doing something good for yourself. Poorly combined meals, meals that combine foods that do not digest well together, provide the immediate punishment of a heavy, stuffed feeling, often fatigue, indigestion, and a grumbly, gassy next few hours. If you tune in to your body following the food that you eat, you will train yourself to combine foods properly. It will be more rewarding to combine foods right than to disregard food combinations or to miscombine intentionally. It takes time, but it works. Just knowing the rules of food combining and agreeing with the theory is not enough to improve health. You must practice what you know.

Knowing the acid/alkaline balance of everything that you eat permits you to enjoy the rewards of an alkaline-based meal or an alkaline food and to understand the discomfort that can be caused by concentrated, acid-forming foods. Eventually you will be choosing many times more alkaline than acid-forming foods.

For a while you will probably refer to this book to discover how a particular food is digested and what its acid/alkaline balance is. However, in a couple of weeks you will identify most of the foods in your diet with ease, rarely referring to the book. Also within a couple of weeks, food combining will become part of your thinking, and you will be looking for more ways to use it.

You may find yourself miscombining many meals at first, intentionally or in error. Don't force this discipline; it must develop because you want it to, not because it was ordered. Meals miscombined from lack of knowledge will eventually become a thing of the past.

Digestibility and alkalinity are really the only two considerations that you will ever need to be concerned about to keep food combining working forever. Remember, if the food you are about to eat is a concentrated acid-forming food (protein, grain, sugar), it is best to combine it with alkaline vegetables to offset the acid influence. Raw vegetable salads are the ideal companions to combine with acid-forming foods. If combining a fresh salad is not appropriate, as with eggs or a dessert, for example, the meal following should be rich in alkaline.

Never follow an acid-forming meal with another acid-forming meal. Follow every meal containing a concentrated protein or starch with an all-vegetable or all-fruit meal. Alternating heavy and light meals will assure a strong alkaline base in the blood. At the same time it will provide a safeguard against overeating and becoming too involved with stimulating and addicting foods. It will also assure easy, frequent elimination because of the roughage, which sweeps the digestive tract clean and tones the whole system.

MORE ABOUT FRUIT

All fruit is alkaline to the body, and it is perhaps the most suitable food for the human digestive process. Fruit is not digested in the stomach, however, and because of the highly fermentable character of fruit, it should be eaten alone. Fruit is best when eaten in the morning. After the long fast of a night's sleep, the evening meal is well out of the way and the fruit will be digested without interference.

Fit for Life

Fruit is classified in four groups as follows.

Acid Fruit	Oranges	**Sweet Fruit**	Bananas
	Grapefruit		Dates
	Lemons		Figs
	Pineapples		Prunes
	Tomatoes		Raisins
	Pomegranates		Papaya
	Strawberries	**Melons**	Honeydew
Subacid Fruit	Apples		Cantaloupe
	Avocados		Crenshaw
	Apricots		Watermelon
	Cherries		
	Grapes		
	Mangos		
	Nectarines		
	Pears		
	Plums		

Fruit Mixtures

Sweet fruits do not mix well with acid fruits, and melons do not mix well with anything. Acid fruits combine with nuts and dairy products. The combination of cheese and fruit is marginally acceptable and certainly better than the protein/starch combination of cheese with crackers or bread.

Correctly, fruit should be eaten at a fruit meal or in between meals and at least four hours after a protein meal. Include fruit in your diet every day to insure against constipation.

MORE ABOUT FAT

Fat combines with starch, a fact that makes food combining achievable. The fat/starch combination allows for baked potatoes with butter and sour cream, bread and butter, avocado sandwiches, and cream on your cereal. Because cooked tomatoes combine with starch, and fat combines with starch, all Italian dishes may be enjoyed as long as meat and/or cheese is not included in the sauce. An avocado sandwich should satisfy your desire for a sandwich when you are so inclined, and a potato with butter, sour cream, bacon, and chives is gourmet fare.

YOUR POINT OF VIEW

Following is a summary of everything you need to know to put food combining to work. Food combining produces superior health because it detoxifies the body. Superior health and terminal disease are on the opposite ends of the same line, and less of one will always produce more of the other.

The case for food combining is indisputable. The logic is clear and sound. If you try it, chances are good you'll like it and find it to be the most important health discovery of your life.

Food Combinations that Agree

Acid Fruit

Combine with:
Nuts
Milk

Green Vegetables

Combine with:
All proteins
All starch

Legumes

Combine with:
Green vegetables

Proteins

Combine with:
Green vegetables

Starches

Combine with:
Green vegetables
Fats

Cooking Rules

1. Do not use aluminum utensils for cooking, as the aluminum can be absorbed into the food. Too much aluminum is very bad for the body.
2. Store oils and fats in the refrigerator.
3. Eat the skins of potatoes and other vegetables.
4. Do not soak legumes in water if you do not use the water. Otherwise you will be throwing away important vitamins and minerals.
5. Vegetables are best raw. Steaming them is next best.

Acid and Alkaline Foods

Acid Cereals

All breads
All flour products
Cookies
Corn
Cornmeal
Crackers
Doughnuts
Dumplings
Macaroni
Noodles
Oatmeal
Rice
Spaghetti

Alkaline Cereals

Buckwheat
Millet

Acid Dairy

All cheese
Butter
Cottage cheese
Cream
Custards
Eggs
Ice cream
Milk—pasteurized, cooked, canned, dried

Alkaline Dairy

Acidophilus
Buttermilk
Koumiss
Raw cottage cheese
Raw milk, raw milk products
Whey
Yogurt

Acid Flesh Foods	*Alkaline Flesh Foods*
Fish	Blood
Fowl	Bone
Meat	

Acid Vegetables	*Alkaline Vegetables*
Artichokes	All other vegetables, especially green leafy
Asparagus tips	
Beans, dried	Cooking destroys alkaline elements
Lentils	
Peanut, filbert, Brazil nut	

Acid Miscellaneous	*Alkaline Miscellaneous*
All alcoholic beverages	Exercise
Candy	Fresh air
Chocolate, cocoa	Honey
Condiments (curry, pepper, salt, etc.)	Laughter
Drugs	Love
Jams and jellies	Sleep
Mayonnaise	Sunshine
Soft drinks	
Stress	
Tobacco	
Vinegar	

Eating Rules for Weight Control

1. Do not eat while standing.
2. Take 30 minutes for every meal.
3. Replace fork after every bite.
4. Eat only at designated, appropriate places.
5. Eat *only;* do no other activity (watching television, talking on the telephone, etc.).
6. Always leave two bites.
7. Take two one-minute intermissions during a meal to slow down the intensity of eating.
8. Delay beginning for one minute while food is in front of you.
9. Eat nothing directly out of a package.

These eating rules are sure to assist you with controlling your weight. If you have weight to lose, Chapter 9 will detail a behavior modification program to make that possible. But whether you are overweight or not, controlling weight is everyone's concern and is practiced by fit people more than by fat people. The extra pound or two that sneaks up on you when you are not careful, every now and again, can be lost most effectively by adhering to these simple eating rules rather than by restricting calories or by fasting. Eating, not food, is the cause of extra weight. Eliminating food will result in temporary weight loss if you only have a pound or two to lose. But that pound or two will come back more regularly if you ignore the eating habits that are the culprits.

MISCOMBINATIONS AND REMEDIES

Food combining should not be looked at as a test of willpower. Food combining is not something you begin Monday morning, like dieting or exercising. Monday morning promises usually weaken your ability to follow through and get the job done. Food combining will develop slowly if you evaluate everything that you eat according to its digestibility and alkalinity.

To Err Is Human

Miscombining is perfectly acceptable as long as you know that you are doing it and know what to do to mend some of the damage. Intentional miscombinations are normal. Indulgences can be planned without retarding your progress or ruining your good record. A pizza or hamburger, a gourmet entree in a very special restaurant, or a special dessert may tempt you for old time's sake for the rest of your life. Don't develop an all-or-nothing attitude about food combining. If you properly combined just one meal a day, you would be improving your health by one-third, and that is a step in the right direction.

There are basically two remedies for miscombined meals. They don't make the miscombinations more acceptable, but they fortify the digestive system so that the irritation will be held to a minimum.

After a miscombined meal, eat a large raw vegetable salad as soon as possible but not later than the next meal. This will speed the elimination of the toxic combination and will refresh the intestines at the same time. Or skip the next meal following miscombining. That will allow the digestive system to rest and to restore strength. With either remedy, the next two or three meals following a miscombined meal should be predominantly alkaline and combined correctly.

As with all things, a price must be paid for miscombining, but the price is manageable, and before long your desire to miscombine will be infrequent and anticipated.

Fruit Cleanses

Food combining contributes so greatly to your health because it keeps the digestive tract healthy, clean, and working the way it was designed to work. Miscombining foods, in addition to producing toxins that the blood distributes throughout the body, clogs the digestive tract. Fruit is one of the best sources of roughage and can be depended on to sweep the digestive system and to add bulk and moisture to the waste product.

Papaya and pineapple are the two most cleansing fruits. If you feel gassy, bloated, or uncomfortable after miscombining, you may want to spend a day eating nothing but fruit to clean the digestive system completely.

Protein/Starch Mixing

There is a theory that the lower end of the stomach is where the acid and stomach enzymes are found, and where churning takes place. The upper part of the stomach, while not actually a separate compartment, is still under the influence of the saliva and will permit the continuation of starch digestion while the lower end digests protein.

Other researchers have suggested that the stomach handles the digestion of foods that have a natural combination of protein and starch by first separating the starch from the protein and digesting the protein while the starch is actually set aside. So it may be possible that each end of the stomach works independently.

In any event, combining protein and starch together in the same mouthful, as with a hot dog and bun, is sure to cause trouble. You may want to keep in mind the stomach sectioning theory if you dine out and are about to miscombine intentionally. If you can save the starch until you have finished eating the protein, you may survive combining the two. Separating the protein and the starch is certainly better than combining everything at once. So, if you cannot resist the freshly baked muffins that your aunt made, and you are planning on roast beef, eat the muffin after you have finished the protein, the longer afterward the better. It would be better, of course, not to risk this combination, but if you must, eat the starch last.

Common Miscombinations

As you begin to practice food combining, many bad combinations will be immediately obvious to you, like meat and potatoes or a ham-on-rye. Other combinations may be just as bad but may not be as obvious. The list that follows may help.

1. *Pizza.* Cheese combines poorly with dough and tomatoes.
2. *Peanut butter and jelly sandwich.* Peanut butter combines poorly with bread; jelly combines poorly with the bread and with the protein in the peanut butter.
3. *Grilled cheese sandwich.* Cheese combines poorly with bread.
4. *Macaroni and cheese.* Cheese is protein, and macaroni is starch.
5. *Cream cheese and bagel or muffin.* Protein combines poorly with starch.
6. *Potato salad.* Eggs in the dressing combine poorly with starch.
7. *Mayonnaise.* The oil combines poorly with eggs.
8. *Mustard.* Fermented condiment that combines with nothing.
9. *Parmesan cheese with spaghetti.* Another protein/starch combination.

10. *Meat sauce with pasta.* Protein/starch combination.
11. *Bacon, lettuce, and tomato sandwich.* Bacon is a fat that combines well with the bread, but tomato is acid and will prevent the digestion of starch.
12. *Bean or lentil soup.* Chicken/beef stock is protein; beans are starch.
13. *Chili with meat.* Chili is starch, meat protein, and tomatoes acid.
14. *Turkey stuffing.* Combines very poorly with turkey.
15. *Gravies.* Flour combined with meat, chicken, or fish stock is poor.
16. *Salad with vinegar or lemon juice and croutons.* Acids combine poorly with starches.
17. *Banana bread.* Fruit and starch combine poorly.
18. *Pies, cakes, cookies, doughnuts.* Sugar ferments starch rapidly.
19. *Fruit pies.* Especially bad combination of fruit, sugar, starch.
20. *Commercial salad dressings.* Usually contain sugar and vinegar; poor.
21. *Coffee with sugar and milk.* Sugar and milk combine poorly.

Uncommon Combinations

The good news is that there are many combinations that are acceptable but not obvious. You will find many unusual but good combinations as you develop the practice of food combining. The following short list will get you started.

1. *Avocado sandwich.* Even though avocado is a protein food, it is mainly a fat. Fats combine well with starch. Use olive oil instead of mayonnaise.
2. *Bacon with starch.* Bacon is a fat. Combine it with breads and with potatoes.
3. *Butter on starch.* Butter is a fat. Combine it with breads, potatoes, corn, cereals, noodles.
4. *Spaghetti with marinara sauce.* Cooked tomatoes combine well with starch.

5. *Ice cream/sherbet*. Not as bad if sweetened with honey and satisfies a sweet tooth.
6. *Cooked cereals with cream*. Not great, but cream is a fat and may be combined with starch.

All or Nothing Gets Nothing

Do not make the mistake of looking at food combining as an all-or-nothing proposition. If you do, it may prove to be nothing for you. Developing fitness and health works in plateaus. If you try to master a level beyond your present ability, you will fail and you may give up. If you decide to make food combining an immediate, permanent way of life, you will fail and you may give up. Remember, changing old habits is a process that requires patience and repetition. Eating properly combined food for good health and a wonderful feeling will keep you on the path to success.

7

Getting Better

During the past ten years a grass roots movement has been growing in the United States away from the traditional medicine toward holistic, natural treatment for the cure of disease.

The holistic health movement is answering the persistent resentment that people feel toward doctors and the high cost of ineffective medical treatment. Modern medicine studies the dead and dying for the treatment of disease. Drugs have become so sophisticated that symptoms can be obliterated in a matter of days. The medical community has become inviolate and often irresponsible. Doctors take complete credit for success but blame failure on fate. The patient is the pawn.

THE CAUSE OF DISEASE

A weakened and overburdened body is the one cause of all disease. Disease is not possible if the nerve energy of the body is vital. Treating disease symptoms with drugs, vitamins, or surgery does not address the problem.

Disappointment with doctors is inevitable. We ask them to make us healthy after we have become unhealthy, and we take the symptoms of deterioration to them to be cured. The symptoms of a disease, whether they be the cough and congestion of a cold or the nausea and fever of a flu, have little to do with the cause.

The body does not deteriorate without reason, nor can it become infected from the outside without invitation. The cause of disease saturates the whole and is manifested in the part. The manifestation is the symptom.

The cause of all disease is a body weakened by physical, emotional, and dietary habits that sap energy from vital functions, causing toxic waste to be retained and then circulated by the blood to poison the feeding, growing cells. In the process of metabolism toxic waste is thrown off by each reproducing cell. When nerve energy is normal broken-down tissue is eliminated as fast as it is produced. But when nerve energy is diminished from any cause enervation of the body results, elimination is repressed, toxins are retained, and the cause of disease is established. Once this accumulation is established it continues until the cause of enervation is removed or a crisis occurs. Disease is the crisis of toxemia.

CAUSES OF ENERVATION

If the body is not enervated, waste will be eliminated and disease will not be possible. To say it differently, superior health is possible only as a result of removing causes of enervation.

If you are reading this chapter to find cures for physical and/or emotional disease, understand this concept of enervation. It is the only hope for cure. If you are reading to improve an already healthy body, study the following causes of enervation, because your health potential and life span can be limited by them.

Overeating

Eating more food than the body can use overburdens every function and produces more waste than the bowels can eliminate within an acceptable amount of time. This saturates the blood with toxic waste, which accelerates enervation, hastening toxemia.

Overeating inflames the lining of the digestive system, producing a toughening of the mucous membranes and a constant infectious secretion that is absorbed by the blood. Toughening of membranes has been cited as a cause of cancer of the colon.

Chronic overeating, of course, leads to obesity, and for the obese individual, enervation is so complete and toxemia so thorough that serious disease and premature death are reasonably predictable.

Improper food combining results in many of the same symptoms as overeating. It is a major cause of enervation because it maintains a toxemic condition once it is established.

Smoking

Smoking tobacco poisons the body. It is possibly the most destructive activity one can pursue without immediate death. Smoking is a leading cause of enervation and contributes to every disease that a smoker develops.

Drinking

Alcohol kills cells in the brain, destroys vitamins completely, paralyzes nerve function, and costs the body vital energy for hours and sometimes days after it is consumed.

Chronic overdrinking will enervate the system so completely that when the inevitable crisis does occur it may be terminal.

Alcohol overstimulates the nervous system to the point of exhaustion. Each time the nerves are overstimulated they weaken, until eventually the nervous system collapses. If alcohol is combined with food, digestive enzymes are destroyed, digestion is incomplete, muscle function is deadened, and waste is retained.

Drugs

Whether prescribed or recreational, taking drugs of any kind destroys healthy energy and replaces it with disguised ability.

Drugs leave behind such unyielding toxins that continuous users of even aspirin always have aches and pains and stiffness. Studies have shown that chronic users of Valium still have residue from the drug two years after discontinuing its use.

Pain pills, sleeping pills, and amphetamines take a large toll on the body for the momentary relief they offer. Their side effects may be dangerous, but they are not nearly as lethal as their main effect.

Coffee and Tea

Caffeine in coffee and tea is a stimulant that robs the body of vital nerve energy, causes dependence, and contributes substantially to providing internal dispair and disease. Caffeine is a serious drug that brings a great deal of misery to many unsuspecting users. It enervates the body to such extent that body temperature is increased after just one cup of coffee or tea.

Sugar

Acting like a drug, sugar stimulates the body with energy borrowed from the body's vital reserve. It is highly addicting and damaging to health. It provides energy without nourishment. Blood sugar skyrockets and plummets. Sugar is so profoundly enervating that sugar junkies who manage to find the courage to give it up demonstrate the signs of withdrawal that drug users display.

Lack of Oxygen

Deep breathing oxygenates the blood and is alkalinizing and energy-building. The tissues need to be supplied with an abundance of oxygen to be healthy. If some kind of physical activity isn't practiced every day that demands deep breathing, cells deteriorate more rapidly, more waste is produced, tissues lose their vitality, and the enervated system can't eliminate the poisons it is producing and becomes toxemic.

Environmental Pollution

Somewhat less enervating than oxygen loss are the pollutants in drinking water, the chemicals in the city air, and the pesticide residual that comes with our food along with the preservatives used in packaging. They all chip away at our vital force to slowly drain our reserve and to enervate the body.

Emotional Conflict

Dissatisfaction is another cause of enervation. The mind influences the body more than any outside influence. Anger, anxiety, fear, envy, and grief will enervate the body and kill as surely as a bullet from a gun.

Injury

The stress from an injury can begin the process of enervation that will continue without much assistance long after the physical damage heals. How many older people have fallen and broken an elbow or a hip, and never recovered? They don't die from the fracture. The injury enervates them so fully that they just fade away.

STRESS IS THE CAUSE OF ALL ILLS

Everything that uses body energy puts stress on the system to get that energy. If more stress is applied than the body can give energy to, it will draw from the energy stores that are reserved for vital functions. Once that vital energy is tapped, the body is enervated and the process of toxemia begins.

Until enough stress is relieved to prevent energy deficit, toxemia will continue to deteriorate every cell in the body until crisis occurs. This is a predictable outcome that becomes more obvious as one grows older and has been toxemic longer.

Children raised in families free of conflict, who eat well, rest properly, and get plenty of exercise, seldom get sick. Conditions don't exist to enervate them, though toxic waste is continually being manufactured in their growing bodies. As they grow older stress is inevitable with exposure to the elements and demands of life. If any of the enervating habits are adopted and added to normal energy drain, the process of enervation and toxemia starts. The young can tolerate the strain of chronic enervation because their tissues haven't been eroding long enough to suffer real structural damage. At some point, however, toxemia will score damaging percentage points.

Resistance to stress is determined by genetic strength and tolerance. Some people who are still alive at the age of 99 attribute their longevity to drinking a quart of whiskey every day since they were 20. Other young, apparently healthy, active people die from cancer and heart attacks in their prime.

Tolerances differ. The 99-year-old man who drank a quart of whiskey every day of his life started out strong. He might have lived a better and even longer life without the whiskey, but in any event, we can safely deduce that first, he was born genetically more tolerant to stress, and second, he had not developed other enervating habits that would have hastened his demise.

THE GERM THEORY

Scientists are constantly looking for the deadly little germs that cause disease.

The environment is full of deadly germs. Every doorknob, public telephone, restaurant plate, and piece of currency has enough germs on it to wipe out a whole neighborhood, if germs could kill. But germs are no threat to a body that isn't enervated and toxemic. A variety of germs pass harmlessly through the body all the time. Only when these germs mix with retained waste in the blood do they incubate and overwhelm the body. Only in a toxic body, too weakened by prolonged enervating habits, can a germ latch on and infect cells. Cells must be degenerating to fall prey to germs, and the immune system must be too sluggish to be on guard effectively.

Stress causes disease, not germs.

NO CURES FOR DISEASE

The body eliminates waste products through the intestinal route, the kidneys, the lungs, and the skin. An enervated system does not have the power to use all those functions effectively, so the ever evolving waste backs up and is redistributed to the cells of all the tissues in the body. This poisoning, or toxemia, cannot continue indefinitely. Eventually, like water pressure building in pipes, if the cause of the enervation or the cause of the building water pressure isn't removed, something has to explode.

The body cannot hold any more poison, and it goes into crisis. The crisis, whether it be labeled flu, pneumonia, nephritis, rheumatism, colitis, hemorrhoids, or cancer, is the body's way of eliminating the infection it has had to deal with for some time. The disease is not the rheumatism or the cancer; the disease is being generated throughout the entire body, and the rheumatism or cancer is only a sign that a greater disorder exists. And it follows that, if you attempt to treat the symptoms as the disease itself, you will prevent the body from eliminating the poisons it cannot eliminate any other way. In other words, if you close off the release valve without removing the source of the rising pressures, the damage sooner or later will be complete and irreversible.

TREATMENT OF DISEASE

The condition basic to all disease symptoms is toxemia.

Crisis will follow crisis, each becoming a more serious expression of emergency until the point of no return is passed and death results.

The following steps can be helpful in curing disease.

1. Eliminate Sources of Enervation

To cure disease, vital energy reserves must be replenished by eliminating habits that enervate. Behavior must be changed if you are sick and you want to get better. Once again, here are the major enervating habits:

1. Overeating
2. Smoking
3. Drinking Alcohol
4. Taking Drugs
5. Drinking Coffee or Tea
6. Using Sugar in Excess
7. Lacking Exercise and Oxygen
8. Living in Stress
9. Feeling Constant Dissatisfaction and Anger

Start at the top of the list, select your habits, and then decide if being well is important enough to you to adjust your patterns. It is not easy to change stressful habits if you are addicted to their stimulation. If one of these habits controls you, the odds are that others do, too.

Make no mistake: if you are struggling with sickness of any kind, the cause is most likely one or more of the above and the cure begins with making changes.

2. Assist Elimination

Once the causes of enervation have been removed, the next step is to assist the body in eliminating stored-up waste by not taking drugs that mask symptoms. When crisis symptoms appear they must run their course.

Physicians are the first to admit that 80 percent of their patients would recover on their own without assistance. Drugs just add more poison to the blood while they reverse the process of elimination.

Eating

If the body is trying to eliminate poisonous waste and to refuel depleted energy reserves, do not burden it with more waste and more work. When you are sick every cell in your body is sick. Absorption of nutrients is checked, and elimination is retarded. Adding food to the body during crisis fuels the disease and delays the recovery.

We can look again to the animal kingdom for examples of basic response to the laws of nature. Wounded or sick animals retreat to sleep and eat nothing until their health improves. Humans have lost most instinct about the natural order of things; our behavior is learned. Eating during a crisis is unnatural.

Work

Your work may be a significant source of stress, keeping you enervated and sick. Even if you love your work and are not able to imagine how it might contribute to making you sick, the responsibility of carrying on and making decisions is counterproductive at a time when you need to conserve all the energy that you can muster.

Rest

Energy conservation is the key to recovering from illness. Whatever your symptoms, rest and perhaps stay in bed until you see signs of improvement.

Hot Baths/Saunas

The skin is the largest organ of elimination, capable of processing more than 30 percent of the body's waste through its pores. Regular, forced sweating is important therapy in all health improvement programs and is essential in a sound plan for health recovery. While you are at home resting and not eating, take two hot baths or saunas a day. Stay in the bath or sauna until you feel your heart beating rapidly. When your heart rate rises there is a point past which your entire body throbs with the beat. This will indicate that your blood is filtering through the liver and kidneys faster and that your temperature is up and you are passing toxins through your skin. While you are in a crisis, do not prolong this stress; leave the bath or the sauna as soon as you feel a rapid heart rate and return to bed and stay warm.

Baths are famous throughout history for curing ailments. Every culture has prescribed hot baths and other water therapy for illness.

Enemas

During recuperation, an enema administered both morning and evening will greatly assist your body in eliminating toxins. Enemas are indispensable in the treatment of disease and should be part of every fasting program. Remember that you are trying to restore vital energy and to eliminate waste. The colon is the depository of most of the waste produced by the body. When you are enervated, the colon lacks the energy to eliminate waste thoroughly. Retained waste is then absorbed by the blood, contributing significantly to the diseased condition.

Generally we are not comfortable talking about the bowels, and consequently most people are ignorant of the functioning and the significance of this vital organ. The bowels are the main source of both health and disease. Waste from all of the organs finds its way into the bowels and must be eliminated without delay. In an enervated condition they need help.

Fresh Air and Sun

Be sure that your rooms are ventilated well. Your lungs are another major organ of elimination, and the toxins thrown off by your breathing should not be trapped in stale, warm air to be breathed again.

The sun has great healing power. If you can, spend some time every day being warmed by the sun without allowing yourself to get burned. It will help restore energy and relax tension.

Healing Crisis

When you feel sick or have any disease symptoms you have

been enervated and toxemic for some time. Now that the crisis has occurred you cannot patch it up again with drugs or with more borrowing. You must flush the waste out, rebuild your strength, and thus cure the disease. Fast to let the body clean and heal itself. However, in the process of cleaning out, you will be eliminating toxins that have stimulated your body before you feel better. Expect that detoxifying will make you feel worse. Think of it as a healing crisis. It is quite normal and is usually a good indication that you are on the mend. Don't give up and go back to mediocre health. Expect this healing crisis and bear with it.

Because of the possibility of a healing crisis, it is wise to consult your doctor about your plans if you have disease symptoms that have affected the heart or the kidneys. In fact, it is a good precaution to let someone know about your fast and have someone follow your progress.

PREVENTING DISEASE

Disease is possible only in a body stressed beyond the point of resistance. Disease is prevented by preventing stress, just as superior health is achieved through deliberate and continuous reduction of stress.

Health and disease are on opposite ends of the same line. Eliminating disease and improving health require similar procedures. Attention must be paid to the same points of stress. It is the same program of improvement; the only difference is in the time that it takes. Building superior health from a healthy foundation is quick, easy, and fun.

Fine-Tuning Health

1. Diet Is the Key

The biggest contribution to the state of one's health comes from good food.

Selecting fresh fruits, vegetables, and high-quality protein is essential to providing the body with the nutrients it needs for growing tissue and for energy. Eat as much "live" food as possible—raw fruits, raw vegetables, nuts, seeds, etc. Avoid packaged and prepared foods because they have undergone too much processing and have lost their vital ingredients.

The body has no specific need for flesh foods. The usable protein from meat, fish, and poultry is generally inferior to that from vegetable sources, and it comes in a form whose life forces are declining and whose waste products alter digestion and rob the body of its vital alkalinity, adding toxins to the blood.

One's diet must be kept clean and highly combustible. Complex carbohydrates in the form of fruits and vegetables are fast burners, and they leave a clean, easily eliminated after product that contributes health-giving alkalinity to the blood. Vegetable carbohydrates should make up 80 percent of your diet.

Minimize protein in your diet. About 1½ ounces of protein a day is used for energy, and more than that leaves the body clogged up with acid waste that constipates. It is true that we need protein foods to provide the amino acids that we cannot manufacture, but the need is small and not a daily requirement. Get protein from nuts, grains, vegetables, and raw dairy products. They are clean foods that don't slow down the system. One protein meal a day, preferably in the evening since it takes so long to digest, is plenty.

Someone once said that you can't be too rich or too thin. To be healthy, you must stay thin. The less body fat that you have, the greater your potential for fitness. Chapter 9 will give you the skills for losing excess weight and keeping it off. Staying thin is an absolutely essential part of being healthy.

Food combining will greatly increase the contribution your diet makes to your health by assuring a higher absorption of nutrients, a minimum of poisonous waste, and significantly less stress on the digestive system. Combining foods properly keeps you fit, svelte, and young.

2. Control Enervating Habits

Enervating habits limit your health potential.

If you are smoking tobacco, you will never achieve a condition of health that can be considered good. Smoking is so damaging to your health that you stand a good chance of dying as a result of it. There are more than 40 known poisons in the smoke of tobacco, any one of which would kill you instantly if injected directly into the bloodstream.

Smoking keeps the body toxic and contributes acid to the blood. It restricts the amount of oxygen going to the tissues and forces cells to retain waste. Smoking is a major cause of enervation and toxemia.

Alcohol, coffee, and tea are all enervating substances that lead to addiction and disease. They sap vital energy with each sip. Better health is possible sooner without their use.

Achieving superior health is a process, not an event. Most enervating habits have some influence on the lives of almost everyone. It is a matter of priorities: for every enervating activity there must be a regenerating activity to counterbalance and to maintain the status quo.

Drug users waste vital energy, whether or not the drugs are prescribed by a physician to cure symptoms or taken to relieve the tension of modern life. They are stressors; just ask any user. If you are taking drugs and seem unable to improve your health through the addition of food combining to your fitness program, you may be sure that the drugs are a major source of enervation and probably will make you sick.

Examine the enervating habits in your life to determine how much strength they are using. Your maximum potential will be limited by your stressing habits.

The emotional stressors are difficult to eliminate without changing large life patterns. But food combining will make you feel better and more satisfied about everything in your life. You will be less anxious, more confident, and better equipped to reorganize your environment. Psychological stress coming from fear, worry, anger, greed, envy, etc., will consume more vital energy than any of the more obvious abuses and will make you just as sick.

3. Exercise

The need for exercise can be interpreted from a number of different points of view.

Exercise is another stress put on the body. The difference between the stress of exercise and the stress that causes the body to become enervated is that the stress of exercise has the effect of cleaning out the body, while the enervating stress loads the body with waste. If exercise is to improve health it must be the aerobic type that forces the heart rate up to within a safe distance of its maximum for a long enough time to result in heavy breathing and profuse sweating. Chapter 8 will explain the latest thinking about exercise.

4. Sleep

Sleep is perhaps the best of all energizers. In addition to restoring vital energy, sleep increases the alkaline base within the body, which, as you know, is vital to the maintenance of life itself.

It is impossible to estimate how much sleep is enough for everyone. Sleep researchers have yet to explain the need for sleep and are beginning to believe that less sleep is better than too much. The amount of sleep you personally need will depend on the extent of stress you must handle during the day. Too much sleep will keep you almost sedated and dulled during your waking hours. Because most people develop regular sleeping patterns, the only way to discover if you may be getting too much sleep is to deliberately cut back ten minutes each day for one week. At the end of one week you will have cut out more than one hour of sleep, and if you have never experimented with your sleeping patterns, don't be surprised to find that you will have more energy and feel better with less sleep.

You will discover as you begin food combining that when your body functions more efficiently you will need less sleep. You may begin waking earlier in the morning. Sleep is a great health giver, but too much sleep keeps a large portion of our population working at half-speed.

With food combining you will need less sleep. Watch for the signs. Don't ignore them.

5. Periodic Fasting

Juice fasting for a week or 10 days will cleanse the body of accumulated waste and will regenerate the cells, the mind, and the will.

After the third day of depriving the body of necessary nutrients it will begin to digest its own tissues. The first tissue the body will feed on will be the most inferior and useless. The cells that are diseased, damaged, dying, or dead will be the first to be burned as fuel. The useless cells of tumors and obstructions are burned next in an attempt to feed on anything that isn't vital to the system. Fat deposits are consumed next, and the body lives very well on its own stores of fuel.

During a juice fast fruit and vegetable juices are consumed for their alkaline healing properties. The liver, lungs, kidneys, and skin, relieved from having to filter incoming products of digestion, will be free to eliminate stored waste and accumulated toxins.

After fasting the body is cleaned out and the digestion of food and the assimilation of nutrients is improved. Enzyme secretion is strengthened, and waste is eliminated freely and efficiently.

Holistic thinking insists that fasting is absolutely necessary in the treatment of any disease, and because the body is fighting waste all the time, the fast is effective insurance against toxemia and is one more step toward achieving superior health.

Learn more about fasting before you undertake your first fast. There are many excellent books that may be found in health sections of bookstores and health food markets.

6. Therapeutic Baths

Water therapies should not be overlooked as valuable assets to every health program. Sitting in a sauna or in a hot tub or taking a hot bath in the evening is more than just relaxing. Overheating therapy, as hot baths are called, has been used by athletes and health enthusiasts for centuries to help maintain fitness and destroy the seeds of illness.

The high temperature of the sauna or hot baths causes the body to develop fever, and fever is one of the body's primary healing forces that is created deliberately to restore health. With fever, metabolism is accelerated, waste is filtered from the blood at a faster rate, toxins are eliminated from the skin by perspiring, and blood is forced to the extremes of all the tissues to bring along nutrients and to sweep away waste.

Hot and cold shower therapy can be used every time you take a shower. It stimulates all the body functions and is especially regenerating for the adrenal glands, the skin, and the circulation. To start, take a warm shower for at least five minutes to warm the body and to draw the blood to the surface. Then switch rapidly to all cold water for 10–15 seconds, making sure to expose your head, chest, back, and legs to the cold. Go back to a warm shower for another five minutes, then again to cold for 15 seconds, to warm once again for five minutes, and finish with cold.

The cold shower is the most famous of the water therapies and is considered a cure-all by some of the early medical philosophers. It improves circulation, increases muscle and skin tone, improves digestion, stimulates the central nervous system and vital organs, and increases the blood count and intake of oxygen. It must be developed gradually, however. The hot and cold shower will prepare you for an all-cold shower. Don't just turn the shower on cold one day and walk in; you may never do it again.

Relative newcomers to the therapy baths are the Jacuzzi and the circulating hot tubs. These hot baths have powerful jets that circulate the water. In addition to providing all the benefits of overheating therapy, the swirling hot water acts as a massage for muscles and joints.

7. Relaxation/Medication

The psychological stresses—worry, anxiety, fear, anger, envy, etc.—take as big a toll in enervating the body and preventing good health as other negative influences. There is no treatment for psychological stress or tension as successful as the daily practice of relaxation/medication procedures. Any of the methods of relaxation takes only 10–15 minutes and should be included at least once a day in the life of everyone who aspires to superior health and longer life.

While all the published methods of relaxation differ somewhat in procedure, the intention of each is to have you focus on the various parts of your body and progressively release the tension in each part. Once you have inventoried and relaxed each of your muscles from head to toes, you then allow your mind to drift away from your body in meditation.

The middle of the morning and the middle of the afternoon are two excellent times for the relaxation process. Each exercise will stabilize your blood sugar, sooth your nerves, and renew energy and self-confidence. After a few weeks of daily relaxation tension, stress, and conflict will be decreased profoundly. The results will astound you. Any book on relaxation will get you started, and before long you will develop your own routine.

8. Massage

Massage is the best of all of the physical therapies. A skilled masseur or masseuse will stretch and lift each muscle in your body, stimulate blood circulation, and strengthen the points of attachment to the bones. Massage will release tension from the muscles, which in turn will immediately lower stress on the body and the demands on the nervous, digestive, and glandular systems.

Massage has been credited with curing every disease imaginable, and rightfully so because it energizes the entire body by physically removing tension and by moving waste from places of deposit.

The therapeutic value of massage just for the skin cannot be overstated. The skin is the largest organ of the body. It works to eliminate more waste than any of the other organs of elimination by discharging impurities through its surface. Massage is the only treatment for dislodging and clearing away the debris that accumulates and ages the skin.

Overall, massage is thought to be the single most effective

therapy for retarding the aging process. Its popularity has been limited by its costs and perhaps by the scarcity of talented practitioners. If you can afford the expense and have the patience to search for talent, a massage at least once a week should become part of your lifestyle.

9. Sun Bathing

The sun has recuperative powers that defy adequate explanation. There is something more to the sun than its brightness and heat. There is a life force quite beyond our understanding.

There is no question that too much sun is dangerous and damages your skin, but the value of regular short sun baths to replenish your reserve of vital energy can be enormous. It is no coincidence that you feel healthy and energized after a vacation in the sun, a day at the beach, or an hour in the backyard. The sun imparts energy and improves your health. A mere half-hour of sun bathing will revitalize you.

PUTTING IT TOGETHER

Achieving superior health is like acquiring wisdom. It is a series of small steps, each of which may seem insignificant.

Including food combining in your fitness program is a dramatic example of improving health with small, simple steps. But don't be fooled by the simplicity. It takes a tenacious, perceptive individual to stick with a program of health improvement before any signs of crisis appear.

It takes time and monotonous attention to detail to understand your body and to improve your health. It doesn't happen at a weekend health resort or simply by joining a health club. It takes at least one year just to interpret the language of your body and then another year to develop meaningful control.

Controlling enervating habits and practicing food combining will contribute unbelievably to your health potential. They will require the most dedication to initiate but will return magic rewards. The other methods of fine-tuning will each contribute smaller amounts to your total picture of health but also with large returns.

There are two effective ways to put this all together. The first, and by far the most effective, is to plunge into everything at the same time. That means beginning with a 10-day fast, abstaining from all enervating habits, exercising lightly, taking therapy baths and saunas, getting massages, etc. This is definitely indicated if you have any disease symptoms. And be alert for a healing crisis even if you are without visible symptoms. The easiest way to give up smoking, or drinking, or poor eating habits is by beginning to change as many of these things in your life as you can at the same time.

The only other effective way to incorporate these fine-tuning points into your life is to feed them in slowly but deliberately over a long period of time, let us say two months. Chapter 10 will give you a design for this approach. It is definitely easier to make changes in habit patterns with a program. It is less dramatic but demands more attention because rewards are drawn out and smaller at each step. Change is more permanent, however, if it is learned and practiced in a precise structured way.

8

Exercise

WHY EXERCISE?

When we start grade school we are urged to exercise. In junior and senior high school we are forced to remove warm, comfortable clothing to dress in skimpy, wrinkled outfits and run around outside or in a gymnasium until a bell relieves us of the misery.

Today exercise is big business. As adults we are intimidated into joining health clubs where we get exercise programs that require a dedication that we know we will never have. We are pressured into buying 50-dollar running shoes to pound our poor bodies on the pavement around the neighborhood. And we all own tennis racquets, hand grips, jump ropes, sweat pants, etc., but nobody ever tells us why we should be so miserable so often. And most of the people who tell us to exercise don't tell us why, nor do they seem to follow their own advice.

Not only do we not know why we are supposed to exercise; we are not quite sure what exercise is or which exercise is best, how long we should do it and how often, what results we should expect, or when and how we should pursue it

With all of this confusion, it is no surprise that most people do not exercise at all, and a great many of those who think that they are exercising are mistaken.

1. Purifying the Body

The most important reason to exercise is to flush the body systems of the poisons that circulate in the blood and then settle in the muscles and organs.

Exercise purifies the body. Under physical strain, the cells in every muscle scream for oxygen and more energy. During real exercise the heart pumps blood more quickly to the muscles to supply their higher demand for oxygen, the lungs breathe deeper in order to oxygenate the blood at a faster rate, and the cells throw off more waste in a violent attempt to burn more fuel for more energy.

During exercise waste is filtered from the blood by the liver, kidneys, lungs, and skin at an enormously high rate so that the blood will have a greater capacity to carry oxygen and fuel to hardworking muscles. This represents the most significant contribution exercise makes to your health. But for this to happen, the exercise must be the kind that raises your heart rate, puts strain on your muscles, and lasts long enough to cause you to sweat well.

2. Sending Oxygen to Extremities

The second reason to exercise is to get oxygen to all the extremities, organs, and the brain. Under the stress of exercise, the blood is particularly rich in oxygen and is forcefully circulated to even the smallest blood vessel. Oxygen is a life giver. Exercise demands more thorough circulation of blood, and as a consequence every cell in the body is bathed in a plentiful flow of oxygen that revitalizes the entire system.

Exercise forces oxygen-rich blood to the fingers, toes, scalp, face, and skin, which are all parts of the body that don't usually have an adequate blood supply and are the first places to show the deterioration of age.

Oxygen-rich blood forced to the brain magically flushes away depression, worry, and anxiety. Researchers have discovered that running is a potent medicine for the mentally ill because it acts to stimulate endorphins, which have a measurable tranquilizing effect on the part of the brain that controls emotions. This is no news to joggers. Ask a jogger who runs more than 30 minutes every day why he does it and he will tell you that he is hooked on the high that running gives.

The extra oxygen forced into the tissues enhances every body function. Digestion becomes easier, elimination more frequent, nails and hair stronger, and water retention minimal. Eyesight improves right after exercise, sleep is improved, and sex is better. In fact, everything that you did before beginning to exercise is improved with exercise.

3. Strengthening the Heart

Exercise eventually lowers the resting heart rate by building a stronger heart muscle that needs to beat less frequently to pump the body's supply of blood.

The heart rate of a well-exercised person is commonly found to be between 40 and 60 beats per minute. The average range found by doctors and considered normal is between 72 and 85 beats per minute.

During exercise the heart muscle is developed just as the abdominal muscles are developed during sit-ups. The stronger the heart, the slower it needs to beat to do the job, and the slower it beats, the longer it will last. Well-exercised people seldom have heart attacks.

The circulating blood and the heavy pounding of the heart during exercise also keeps the arteries clean and healthy. Deposits that can form on the walls of the arteries and are responsible for arteriosclerosis and other heart malfunctions are washed away by the rushing blood and pulsating arteries. The entire cardiovascular system is kept strong and clean with exercise, prolonging its effective life.

4. Controlling Weight

Exercise is the most effective method for controlling weight. Well-exercised people are not fat, and though they are aware of the caloric value of foods, they are never obsessed by this factor.

There is a wonderfully logical reason why thin people don't gain weight eating everything that they want why and why fat people don't ever seem to lose weight, though they carefully eliminate every unnecessary calorie.

The body chemistry of a fat person has been changed as the result of being fat so that more fat is stored from fewer calories. The thin person has a normal body chemistry that naturally stores no fat, even when calorie limits have been exceeded. Exercise can provide the body chemistry that will fight fat.

The storage of fat is a natural body function. Sixty to 70 percent of the energy needed by the muscles come from fat; the rest of the energy comes from glucose. Almost half of a well-proportioned body is a muscle, and that muscle burns 90 percent of all the calories that the body uses. The body is prepared to burn fat to provide energy to the muscles, but it is also capable of storing fat in the muscles if those muscles aren't exercised to capacity.

As we grow older our level of activity decreases. The long, lean muscles of youth are no longer used to capacity, and they slowly begin to shorten and soften with the storage of fat. Before any fat can appear on the outside of muscles it must first fill the muscles to their capacity. Overweight people are not able to diet away their extra weight and to keep it off because their muscles are so thoroughly saturated with fat.

To avoid the struggle of gaining and losing 10 pounds periodically throughout your life, you must make your muscles lean so that the circulating fat and the small stores of body fat will be burned for energy and not allowed to marble the muscles and slow the metabolism. The only way to keep the muscles lean and free of fat deposits is through exercise or prolonged starvation. Unfortunately for the overweight, after the subcutaneous fat is lost the real job of losing the intramuscular fat begins and may take a year or two of careful eating and continuous exercise to complete.

WHAT IS EXERCISE?

Do not confuse work with exercise!

For physical activity to be exercised and to accomplish the four basic goals of exercise, it must be aerobic. Aerobic exercise is a steady exercise that demands an uninterrupted output from your muscles for a minimum of 20 minutes at a heart rate that is 80 percent of its capacity.

If the physical activity or uninterrupted stress does not reach your maximum capacity for at least 20 minutes, it is not exercise. And if an aerobic exercise is not practiced at least four times a week, it will not achieve the above goals.

Housework, gardening, shoveling snow, picking up bags of cement all day, and digging ditches are all work, but they are not exercise. They use the muscles, they even strain the muscles, but without uninterrupted stress accomplished by the rapid circulation of oxygen-rich blood, the strain of work will drain energy, will fill the muscles with acid that makes them stiff and sore, and will be just another stress that erodes your health.

Many athletic activities that don't qualify as exercise are wonderful sports to enjoy. Tennis is a game that cannot be considered exercise unless it is highly competitive and played for two or three hours a day, every day. Weight lifting is not exercise; neither is stretching or calisthenics, golf or downhill skiing, racquetball, handball, or squash. They exhaust your body and health rather than improve it.

Any physical activity that is continuous for a minimum of 20 minutes and requires the heart rate to accelerate to 80 percent of its capacity (and no more than 85 percent) is aerobic exercise. With aerobics all your muscles become lean and toned, no matter which muscles bear the burden of the exercise.

Running and jogging are the best aerobic exercises. Walking can be aerobic and is the first choice for people who can't take the enormous physical abuse of running. Jumping rope is a top aerobic exercise, as are steady bicycling, rowing, dancing, roller skating, etc. More about each one later.

HOW AEROBICS WORK

The value of aerobic exercise for eliminating toxins through sweating, deep breathing, and rapid blood circulation is easy to understand and consistent with the traditional view of exercise. Powering oxygen to the tissues, stimulating hormones, and strengthening the heart, arteries, and lungs are the obvious benefits from continuous stress exercise. Now, thanks to the pioneering work of Kenneth Cooper and Covert Bailey, and the hours and hours of sweat and measurement endured by the dedicated volunteers contributing to research of this book, there may be a better understanding of what exercise is and how it is best undertaken. The continuous stress of aerobic exercise is proving to be even more effective in developing superior health because of the actual function of the muscles being used.

Seventy percent of the energy needs of muscle is met by fat and only 30 percent by glucose. Glucose is like the kindling that burns easily and quickly in a fireplace. Fat is like the heavy, slow-burning logs that need some help to get started but then burn hot and long once started. Glucose supplies immediate energy to the muscles, and fat supplies the energy for the long pull.

All cells in the body require some form of energy fuel. With the exception of muscle cells, the energy requirement of the cells of the body stays relatively constant whether those cells are at the peak of their activity or they are resting. Muscle cells, on the other hand, will demand as much as 50 times more energy going from a resting state to sudden movement. Energy fuel comes to all cells from the blood, but because the muscle cells have to draw so much energy on such short notice, they are equipped with special enzymes that metabolize the nutrients delivered by the blood quickly and in huge volume. Like amplifiers, these muscle enzymes enable the muscles to burn a lot of calories quickly.

With muscle accounting for as much as 50 percent of the body and responsible for burning 90 percent of the calories, the muscle enzymes that enable the muscles to burn all those calories play a prominent role in the state of our health.

These metabolizing muscle enzymes are contained within muscle cells in sacks called mitochondria. Only the muscle cells possess mitochondria. It has been proved over and over again that regular aerobic exercise increases the number of mitochondria within individual muscle cells as well as the amount of metabolizing enzyme within the mitochondria.

If muscle is not used to capacity, it stores fat. As the fat takes the place of the muscle, mitochondria and muscle enzymes are lost, along with the facility to burn calories. You will remember that 90 percent of the calories are burned by the muscles. They are calorie-burning machines. If they are saturated with fat, they lose their burning function.

Aerobic exercise is a slow-and-steady kind of stress placed on the body, 50 percent of which is muscle. At the start of an aerobic exercise glucose acts as kindling to get the energy fire going to meet the increasing demand of the muscles for fuel. As the demand increases the burning of calories must increase to meet the demand. As glucose supplies become exhausted, and as the demand for more fuel continues to increase, fat begins to meet the demand and the remaining glucose is reserved for an emergency in which a sudden burst of muscle action may be needed.

Fat accumulates in the muscles before it accumulates outside the muscle, where it is noticed as extra weight. And fat is drawn from the muscle to be used for energy before it is taken from the adipose tissue surrounding the muscle.

Aerobic exercise burns fat from the muscles for its own energy at the same time that it is increasing the amount of enzymes within the muscles that make that fat burning possible.

A continuous cycle of burning fat and producing fat-burning enzymes keeps the well-exercised body resistant to fat storage. The cycle becomes vicious, however, for the individual who is out of shape and is becoming fat. The ability to use fat for energy decreases as the muscles lose their tone; energy comes mostly from blood glucose as the muscles lose their ability to burn fat. Blood glucose is limited and will be exhausted quickly should the body be put under any physical stress, stimulating hunger and producing more fat.

THE FAT GET FATTER

Burning blood glucose instead of fat for energy is the beginning of a chain of events for a fat person that leads to the storage of more fat from less food and makes losing weight nearly impossible.

When glucose is burned for energy in place of fat the supply of glucose becomes depleted and a mild condition of hypoglycemia develops, causing some degree of fatigue, irritability, and hunger. In order to replenish the blood glucose, whatever is eaten will be converted to glucose, and if carbohydrates are eaten, blood glucose levels will soar. Whenever glucose enters the bloodstream the pancreas matches it with the secretion of insulin. Without insulin, blood glucose cannot be used by the cells. No matter how much glucose is circulating in the blood, insulin must pave the way and chemically unlock each cell in order for the glucose to be utilized as fuel.

As one gets fat the muscles lose their sensitivity to insulin and won't unlock cells as readily to accept glucose. Glucose levels remain high after eating, and when the muscle cells reject the glucose it finds a waiting home in the fat cells. Inside the fat cells glucose is converted to glycerol, and glycerol combined with three molecules of fat becomes triglyceride. Triglyceride is what fat is made of.

So, as the muscles lose their tone they get fat. Fat muscles resist burning fat for energy and burn blood glucose almost exclusively, which sooner or later exhausts the supply and produces an emergency hunger. Any carbohydrate food consumed in response to the low blood sugar alarm is immediately turned into blood glucose, which the muscles will not accept because of their insensitivity to insulin. High levels of blood glucose are quickly absorbed by the fat cells, and the fat get fatter on fewer and fewer calories, trapped in a cycle seemingly with no end.

Anyone who is out of shape and getting fat must adjust eating behavior to limit the exposure to food. Begin with the practice of food combining to unclog the system and then find an aerobic exercise that will slowly and steadily burn intramuscular fat.

LONGER, NOT HARDER

Exercise that doesn't cause the heart rate to reach 80 percent of maximum is called *anaerobic*, which means without oxygen. Exercise that exceeds 80 percent of the maximum heart rate is also anaerobic because the lungs and heart will not be able to supply the oxygen demanded by the muscles.

Eighty percent of the maximum heart rate is called the *training rate*. Exercise that doesn't reach the training rate uses precious glucose for fuel and is anaerobic. Exercise that exceeds the training rate also uses glucose exclusively for fuel. Anaerobic exercise cannot supply the muscles with enough oxygen to burn fat, nor can it promote the creating of more fat-burning emzymes.

The primary job of blood glucose is to fuel the brain. It is the only nourishment that the brain uses, and if it is withheld, the brain will lose consciousness and eventually die. The liver can convert protein into glucose in the event that it isn't supplied otherwise. Anaerobic exercise that exceeds the training rate quickly exhausts blood glucose and forces the body to consume its own muscle protein to keep the brain fed. If the anaerobic exercise is strenuous enough, protein cannot be converted to glucose fast enough, and unconsciousness will result. If strenuous anaerobic exercise short of causing a glucose blackout is continued, muscles will be stripped away, leaving more room for fat and fewer fat-burning enzymes. Just as with anaerobic exercise that is below the training rate, overexercising also works to promote fat storage and chemical imbalance.

As one exercises aerobically more frequently, the muscles become more adept at using oxygen and burning fat. If you are in a bigger hurry to get into better shape, exercise longer, not harder. If you exercise above your training rate, you will be defeating your purpose while undermining your health. The heart is a muscle too, and it is quite possibly the most valuable muscle in the body. If you force your body to make glucose from protein, the heart may suffer the biggest loss. Weekend tennis players and occasional raquetball players have exceptionally high incidents of heart attacks and strokes.

TRAINING HEART RATE

Your training heart rate is 80 percent of your maximum heart rate, which is determined by your age. For people of age 20 or younger, the maximum has been estimated to be 200 beats per minute. Scaling down from there, the maximum heart rate of a 50-year-old person is estimated to be 150 beats per minute. It would seem that the maximum heart rate of a conditioned athlete would be higher than a beginning jogger, which is not the case. The beginner will reach his maximum long before the athlete, however, and the out-of-shape jogger may be forced to slow down to a walk to keep his heart beating at the training rate.

The table on page 108 will give your maximum heart rate for your age and the recommended training rate of 80 percent. Training rates are calculated on resting heart rates. The average resting heart rate for men is 72 beats per minute, and for women it is 80. Those of you who are in better-than-average shape will have lower resting rates. Three columns have been included in the chart to indicate the recommended training rates of 50, 55, and 60 beats per minute.

The formula for arriving at your training heart rate is:
[Maximum minus Resting] × 65 Percent + Resting =
Training Heart Rate

Example: You are 38 years old with a resting heart rate of 65 beats per minute. Maximum heart rate for anyone 38 is 184 beats per minute. 184 minus 65 equals 119. Sixty-five percent of 119 equals 77.4; 77.4 plus your resting heart rate of 65 equals 142.4. Your training heart rate would be 142–143.

The heart rate table gives you an opportunity to see how training rates compare and how yours will decrease as you get

| | | 80% of Maximum at Resting Heart Rate | | | | |
Age	Maximum Heart Rate	80	72	60	55	50
20	200	158	155	151	149	147
22	198	157	154	150	148	146
24	196	155	153	148	147	145
26	194	154	151	147	145	144
28	192	153	150	146	144	142
30	190	152	149	145	143	141
32	189	151	148	144	142	140
34	187	150	147	143	141	139
36	186	149	146	142	140	138
38	184	148	145	141	139	137
40	182	147	144	140	138	136
45	179	144	142	137	136	134
50	175	142	139	135	133	131
55	171	139	136	132	130	129
60	160	132	129	125	123	121
65+	150	126	123	119	117	115

into better shape and your resting heart rate decreases. Use the formula to calculate your training rate if it isn't in the table, but remember that these calculations are based on averages and you may very well not fall exactly in the center of the average. The purpose of the training rate is to give you a tool for pacing yourself so that your exercise will not be wasted at a speed that is too slow or too fast. As you develop aerobics you will have to stop during your exercise from time to time to take your pulse. It is annoying and disruptive to stop an aerobic exercise to count your heartbeat, so you will want to begin to get a feel for your training rate and then check your pulse at the finish. Use these criteria to develop your feel:

1. Stay ahead of your breathing. Do not struggle for breaths.
2. Push your exercise; do not let your exercise pull you. Do not feel fatigue.
3. Be able to carry on a conversation while exercising. Do not overexercise.
4. Breathe with full lung capacity. Do not underexercise.

HOW TO TAKE YOUR PULSE

You can find your pulse most easily on the thumb side of your wrists and on the inside of the two long muscles that run up the front of your neck.

Using the second hand of a watch, count the number of times your heart beats for six seconds, then multiply that number by 10 to arrive at your heartbeat per minute. At first you will count whole numbers like 6, 7, 8 during the six-second period, which will be 60, 70, or 80 beats per minute when you multiply by 10. Practice taking your six-second heart rate so that you will be able to count half-beats and quarter beats to get a more accurate pulse when you multiply by 10. If you count eight beats, for instance, and the eighth beat comes a bit before the sixth second, you will know that your heart is really beating faster than 80 beats per minute, and you may want to count 8.5 beats to arrive at a more accurate 85 beats per minute.

The six-second pulse is the best method for finding your heart rate while exercising. You will have to stop exercising to take your pulse, and any count longer than six seconds will be inaccurate, because as soon as you stop, your heart rate goes down quite rapidly.

You can also use the six-second pulse to find your resting heart rate. However, since the resting rate is used to calculate your training rate, it may be safer to use the traditional 15-second pulse or 30-second pulse to be more accurate. Take your resting pulse a number of times during the day until you clearly see your resting rate emerge. Drinking a cup of coffee or being startled by a loud noise will cause an increase in your pulse rate. If one number doesn't repeat itself after taking your resting pulse six or seven times during the course of a day, add all the rates together and divide by the number of times you took your pulse to find the average.

CAUTION!

If you are over the age of 40 and you are not accustomed to aerobic training, or if you have ever had heart, kidney, or lung problems *do not* begin an aerobic exercise program until you have consulted your doctor and have had a *stress electrocardiogram.*

Exercising at 80 percent of your maximum heart rate places serious stress on your heart, and if you are in a high-risk area, it would be foolish to chance that kind of risk without an OK from your doctor. Unlike regular electrocardiograms (EKGs) that record the heart function while the patient is lying still, stress (EKGs) monitor the heart under stress as the patient steadily increases his output on a treadmill. If your physician finds any abnormalities in your heartbeat under the stress of exercise, he may advise aerobic exercise anyway, but he will certainly want you to work up to your 80-percent training rate slowly over a long period of time. Or, he may not want you to exceed 70 or 75 percent.

CHOOSING AN AEROBIC EXERCISE

The major consideration when choosing an aerobic exercise is to find one that will permit you to exercise at your training heart rate. Selecting an exercise that is no strain at all, like a slow walk through the meighborhood will be obvious. But you will be amazed at how easy it is to exercise beyond your training rate and even beyond your maximum.

To repeat: exercising above or below your training heart rate is worse than not exercising at all, especially if you gain weight easily.

Before you buy an exercise outfit, buy a wristwatch with a second hand. Know your resting heart rate and memorize your training rate before you lace up your sneakers and be prepared to reach it with half the exercise you had planned and in one-fourth of the time.

Know a few things about real exercise if you are just beginning. You will increase your chances of successfully putting together an exercise program that you will continue if you know the following facts.

1. Set a more distant goal. More than three-quarters of all beginners quit after the fourth outing.
2. Set a time of day to exercise, like an appointment. It is easier to exercise at the same time every day.
3. Plan to exercise no fewer than three days a week. Work toward a goal of five or six days if you want to make real progress.
4. Develop more than one aerobic exercise. One indoor and one outdoor exercise will see you through the seasons and help you maintain your interest.
5. Exercise is hard work, and until your body becomes conditioned, it is painful. After you get into shape the endorphins pumped to your brain will keep you coming back forever.
6. An overambitious program must fail. Start simply, but have a plan that leads you to goals.

7. It will take you six months of exercising every other day to notice any results. Be prepared to be patient but stay motivated.

Aerobic exercise will make you feel so good after you get conditioned to it that you will crave it if you miss a scheduled time. Develop positive addiction to exercise: exercise the same time each day; don't exceed your training heart rate; transcend the pain; and gradually build up. Also, it is better to exercise alone. Aerobic exercise is not competitive; it is personal, like meditation. Even if you choose an aerobic dance class as one of your exercises, disregard your neighbor and socialize before and after the class. If you are going to put in time every day or every other day, you may as well learn to love exercise, and you will, if you do it alone and know what you are doing.

AEROBIC EXERCISES

Jogging/Running

Running is the king of aerobic exercise. It is natural movement. Once any infant animal is confident about walking, running then becomes the preferred way to move. The monotony of a running stride is hypnotic, mind-expanding, and truly addicting.

There isn't an athlete in the world who doesn't depend on running to keep in shape. It uses the lungs to full capacity and supplies the body with enormous amounts of oxygen for burning fat and for eliminating.

Running is the best exercise for conditioning the heart and the lungs and for improving circulation. Unfortunately, however, it is not for everyone. If you are fat, you should not run, and if you are over 50 and underexercised, you most definitely should not begin a running program. Women, too, should consider the drawbacks before beginning a running program. The jolt of hitting the ground a few thousand times a mile can be damaging to the breasts and the uterus. I personally advise against it. The treadmill and stationary bicycle are better choices.

The damaging side effects of running outweigh the benefits for many people. Running injures the feet, the knees, the shins, and the lower back. And for many runners, it keeps them nursing pulled muscles and stiff necks. Running may well be considered punishing from many points of view. Because running tightens your muscles, it is extremely important to stretch your legs and back thoroughly before and after you run. The salespeople in any of the athletic shoe stores can recommend good stretching programs.

Equipment

Buy your running shoes in a store that specializes in them. Don't ask salespeople about which pair to buy; try on *every* pair and buy the pair that is the most comfortable and that makes you feel agile. If you don't feel good, you won't keep running, and if the shoes aren't comfortable from the moment that you put them on, they will never be comfortable and may injure your feet. Running shoes have come a long way from the sneaker. They are incredible. Buy the best that you can afford, and again, take no one's advice. Listen to your own body.

Do not wear too much clothing when you run. Shorts and a T-shirt are good in temperatures that are as low as 40°F. If you need more warmth, wear lightweight cotton instead of bulky sweats or polyester blends. Sweats get too heavy after they absorb perspiration, and the blends have a way of making your perspiration feel cold and chilling.

Don't forget the most important piece of running equipment— your wristwatch. It will take you awhile to get your heart rate up to the training level once you begin to run. After you have reached your level, do not go above or below it for a minimum of 20 minutes. Run longer if you wish, but slow your pace down as you tire to maintain your training level.

Walking

Walking is an excellent exercise for older people and for those who are overweight. It uses the same muscles as running uses, and it is far less punishing to the skeleton.

Use your watch to find a pace that maintains your heart rate at 80 percent of maximum, and once you reach that, concentrate on breathing deeply and walk for at least 20 minutes. You may want to try brisk walking to get in shape for running. You will know when to switch over when you can no longer walk fast enough to maintain your training heart rate.

Swimming

It is said that swimming uses all the muscles in the body. It is an excellent aerobic exercise for the cardiovascular system, but it tends to conserve fat supplies to keep the body warm.

Long-distance swimmers have long, well-defined muscles, but not without fat. So if one of your exercise goals is to become lean, swimming may not do it for you.

One young woman I know loves the solitude of swimming so much that she worked out a combination of exercises so that she can enjoy her swimming and, at the same time, be assured of top conditioning. She runs for 15 minutes from her house to the YMCA pool, swims for 30 minutes, and after a steam bath and shower she walks back home. That's the best of everything.

Roller Skating, Ice Skating

Skating is a good aerobic exercise if you maintain your training heart rate for at least 20 minutes.

Cross-Country Skiing

This has all of the benefits of running without the trauma of pounding your feet on the ground. Unless you live in snow country and have a lot of time on your hands, cross-country skiing may be considered a sport for which your daily aerobics get you in shape.

Cycling

Cycling can be an excellent form of aerobic exercise if you set out to ride nonstop for many miles. If you are willing to work at cycling, you can take your pulse without stopping and should theoretically be able to get a perfect workout. The only drawback to outdoor cycling, and it is a big one, is the automobile exhaust fumes that you are forced to inhale at a time when your demand for oxygen is at its peak. The harm done by powering petrochemical waste into the deepest cells of the lungs can never be offset, adding toxins to the body that may never be eliminated.

Stationary Bicycling

Stationary bicycling is an excellent indoor aerobic exercise that requires a sizable investment. It is great for those who are overweight and out of shape, because the tension can be adjusted on the wheel to make peddling harder or easier, and the speed with which you pedal can also be adjusted to pinpoint your training heart rate accurately. Most stationary bicycles wind up in the garage after sitting in a corner of the bedroom unused for about a year. Try to borrow one before you buy to see if you like it. The only people that I know who manage to continue cycling indoors either set the bike up in front of the morning news on television or listen to music with headphones.

It will take quite awhile to get your heart up to speed, so don't begin your 20 minutes until you know that your heart is up to your training rate. And to make the exercise complete you must concentrate on breathing deeply; for some reason the stress doesn't stimulate the lungs to take in more oxygen.

Treadmill

This is one of the best indoor aerobic exercises. It is easier on the body than running, with all the same benefits. The treadmill is a major piece of exercise equipment, however, and is usually found only in health clubs. If you belong to a health club that has a treadmill, try it a few times. Once you get over feeling like a hamster running to go nowhere, it is easy to find a pace that will give you a perfect workout.

Jumping Rope

This is one of the all-time great conditioning exercises, but it's very hard to master and very hard on your body.

The proper way to jump rope is to jump one foot at a time. It will take you months of practice to jump for even one minute without missing. For the beginner, jumping for one minute may drive the heart rate to the limit. Be careful with this exercise.

If you can get through the frustration of learning to jump rope, it is an aerobic exercise that can go anywhere you go and be practiced in the smallest space. Boxers, who are the best-conditioned athletes in the world, rely on the jump rope for developing endurance and coordination. Buy a leather one from a sporting goods store. They are inexpensive and are made with ball bearings in the handles to assist your timing.

Running in Place

This is another good aerobic exercise for those who are overweight and out of shape. Exertion can easily be adjusted by how high you lift your legs. Find a soft surface to run on. Running in place is another exercise that takes a toll on the body and should not be done every day.

Jumping Jacks

This is a good aerobic exercise that uses the upper body better than running in place or jumping rope. It is hard on the body and should be alternated every other day with another exercise that isn't as jarring to the body.

Dancing

Aerobic dance classes are popping up everywhere. They are as good as the instructor and can be terribly punishing if the pace is too fast and the routines are too complicated.

Aerobic dancing is really stretching and pulling muscles to music. The music is infectious disco or rock music that makes you want to move as soon as you hear it, and the exercises begin with warm-ups and accelerate to exhaust every major muscle group in the body.

The music hypnotizes, so it is easy for the group to be led into a pace that will exceed your maximum heart rate. The movements are sometimes violent and punishing to the muscles. The experienced aerobic dancer seems almost proud to be able to endure an hour or more of the most physically abusive movement short of being a tackle in the National Football League.

You will get the best exercise if you do aerobic dancing in your own house, alone, and at your own pace. Instruction books and special aerobic dance records are available, but you may have to attend a few classes to learn the procedure. Most health clubs now have aerobic dance classes, as do the YMCAs and community recreational facilities. If you are a beginner, any group you join will be dancing at a pace beyond your capacity, so be very careful to go slowly beyond your capability, so be very careful to go slowly so as not to exceed your training heart rate or the limits of your muscles.

In aerobic dance class, it is difficult to work at your own pace and not to compete with the group. That's the catch that makes an aerobic dance class unsuitable for most people. Keep up with the group, and you may find yourself unable to bend over far enough to put on your shoes or unable to lift your arms high enough to wash your hair for a week.

ANAEROBIC EXERCISE

Anaerobic exercise is really not exercise at all in the sense of conditioning the body and should be thought of as a recreational sport.

Again, don't confuse work with exercise.

Tennis, racquetball, handball, squash, weightlifting, baseball, group volleyball, etc., will tire you out before they condition you. There isn't enough sustained effort to oxygenate the tissues to burn fat or to strengthen the heart. The effort used in those sports usually exceeds the maximum heart rate at times and then underuses the heart at other times. Don't let heavy sweating and exhaustion fool you into thinking that work is exercise.

9

The Control of Weight

Those who are physically fit are more concerned about their weight than anyone who has a weight problem, and they demonstrate more personal management over their eating. Fat people seem to think that the other guy is just blessed.

The truth is that those who are fit need information about weight control even more because they are the people who work at keeping those extra two pounds out of sight. And without some tools with which to work, controlling weight can become tricky and worrisome and usually means always gaining, and then losing, and then gaining again.

This chapter is not another scheme for weight loss. It is a real, workable method for controlling weight to take the pressure off and to end the worry about getting fat.

EATING IS THE PROBLEM, NOT FOOD

To begin with, it is extremely important to understand that food doesn't make anyone fat. Eating makes people fat. It is a ridiculous notion to try to control food to control weight and, incidentally, is the reason why few people are successful at losing weight on a diet. Trying to control food to control weight will turn into a monster that will keep you afraid of food and vulnerable to the chance of gaining weight that you will not be able to lose.

Eating habits are learned. Learning bad eating habits is the foundation for obesity, and often those bad eating habits are learned from overweight parents and later expanded during times of stress and disappointment. Learning good eating habits will become just as automatic, especially if a healthy relationship with food already exists and your eating is not out of control.

Food combining will give you an immediate edge in controlling your weight. You will probably lose weight as soon as you begin to use food combining, and if you are the kind of person who has trouble keeping weight on, be assured that when your body adjusts to processing and eliminating food more efficiently, you will gain back any weight that you need. You may find, as I did when I began, that less weight makes you feel better, and you may not want to gain any back. In any event, the boost that food combining will give you and the following habit-shaping tips will put you easily in control of your eating and of your weight.

TAKE 30 MINUTES TO EAT EVERY MEAL

Of all the things that cause overweight, eating too fast is the most significant. Almost without exception, those who are overweight eat more food than they want to because they eat faster than their body can process the food.

We are equipped with a signaling function called an *appestat*. Like a thermostat, the appestat will cue the brain when the body needs fuel or when enough has been consumed. We respond by feeling hungry and thinking about food or by feeling satisfied and losing interest in food. The appestat signal to stop eating is easily missed because it takes at least 20 minutes after beginning to eat for the appestat to be triggered.

Make it a rule whenever you sit down to eat a meal to spend a minimum of 30 minutes to eat. Give your appestat ample time to signal when to stop eating. If you get the full signal, quit. Listen to your body. Your interest is in feeling satisfied. Your appestat will keep you thin forever.

If you know that eating fast is your habit, you will have to train yourself to slow down. It's easy. Just make a strict point of spending 30 minutes eating at each of your next 10 meals. That should fix a new habit. It doesn't take long to establish habit patterns if they are practiced at first without deviation. For the next 10 meals, do whatever you must to spread out your eating over 30 minutes. Take a timer to the table for the first couple of meals if you think it may help, cut your food up into tiny pieces, chew each bite 50 times, don't take another bite until everything in your mouth is swallowed and the taste is gone (taste lasts only about one minute), eat with your other hand, use chopsticks—do anything you can think of to get the feeling of eating a meal for 30 minutes for 10 meals. And always, always put down the fork after each bite. Eating slowly is enjoyable; just take the time to find out.

EAT ONLY AT DESIGNATED PLACES

Just follow this rule, and you will greatly decrease your chances of *ever* becoming fat. Permission to eat must be confined to the smallest area possible. Eat only at places designed specifically for eating. There may be many designated places to eat in your day: the dining room table, the kitchen table, a restaurant table, a picnic table, on your lap at a buffet, etc.

Make it your own private rule never to eat while standing. If you observe this rule, most of the job is done. Just think of the unnecessary calories consumed thoughtlessly while you are standing and you give yourself license to eat anything anywhere. With that much leeway you stand a very good chance of getting fat soon, if not sooner.

Remember, controlling weight is controlling eating. Control is discipline—it must be learned, you are not born with it. Minimize your exposure to calories by controlling your eating places. Eating on your feet is the biggest trap, but eating while in bed will eventually destroy you, and so will eating in the car, on the living room couch, at your desk, etc. If you develop a pattern of eating at inappropriate places, those places will soon cue you to eat even though you may not be hungry. Buying popcorn or a candy bar at the movies often enough will cause an association between food and films. At some point you will not be able to go to the movies without either buying candy or popcorn, and you will have begun the losing battle of trying to control food to control your weight. For some people, merely walking through the front door of their houses cues them to go straight to the kitchen to get something to eat. Don't let that happen to you. Don't make food your enemy by permitting yourself to eat it anyplace that you find it.

EAT ONLY: NO OTHER ACTIVITY

Do not eat in front of the television set! Eventually television will make you fat. Habit patterns are easy to form. Eat a handful of goodies at a time in front of the television, and without your knowing it, television will cue you to think about food every time you sit in front of it. Many smokers are cued to lighting a cigarette when the telephone rings or when they smell coffee. Pairing eating with another activity will make you vulnerable to eating when you are not hungry, which will be your undoing.

When you eat, give eating your undivided attention. You will develop a nice relationship with food and will never feel deprived. If you eat while doing something else, in addition to setting up a cuing system, you will eliminate the satisfaction that comes from eating, and you may eat more than you need or even more than you want.

This rule, combined with eating only at appropriate eating places, will serve you well in eliminating external cues to eat and will allow you to respond to your natural internal communication without being a slave to artificially programmed desire.

TAKE TWO INTERMISSIONS

Eating is an intense activity. Digestive juices flow, the heart beats faster, blood pressure goes up, and the body goes to work. We have all seen the movies of the frenzied eating of sharks and of lions tearing apart their prey. All animals speed up when they eat. We need to slow the momentum of eating to be prepared to stop when the appestat signals.

In your mind's eye divide each of your meals into three segments. About 10 minutes after starting, push your chair away from the table. Adjust your sitting position. Take a deep breath and exhale slowly and relax for at least one minute. You will lower your heart rate and blood pressure and diminish the intensity of eating. Then go back to eating slowly and replacing the fork after each bite.

During the second intermission it will be time for your appestat to signal that sufficient food has been consumed. Again, push your chair away from the table and take a deep breath and exhale slowly. Now your diaphragm should be touching your distended stomach, and you must analyze how you feel and decide whether you are full. If you decide you haven't had enough to eat, relax a minute or two and go back to eating very slowly and be alert for the signal to stop. If you decide at your second intermission that you feel full, pay attention to that feeling and stop eating. For some, this may be a big decision. Risk it. Stop eating and leave food behind. The worst that can happen is that you will be hungrier for your next meal, and being hungry is far more comfortable than being stuffed.

If you watch really thin people eat, you will notice that they spend more time at a meal not eating than eating. They have to tell restaurant waiters four or five times not to take their plates away. They haven't developed the frenzy of eating. By insisting that we take at least two formal intermissions during each meal, we will physically slow down the intensity of eating and will psychologically reaffirm our intention not to get carried away.

DELAY BEGINNING

Don't begin a meal with the momentum of the activity that preceded it. When you get to the table, wait for one minute before you begin to eat. This will set a relaxed mood that will prevail throughout the meal. Together with taking two intermissions, delaying the start of a meal for one minute will give you time to compose yourself and to plan how you will be eating your meal.

When you were a child you probably were scolded for coming to the dinner table and immediately reaching for something to eat before everyone was seated and served. The time you had to wait before being permitted to eat slowed you down and forced you to get comfortable. You began eating feeling more relaxed, and consequently you ate less and digested food better.

Don't miss this opportunity to calm down before you eat. You will feel better, enjoy your food more, and minimize your chances of becoming fat.

LEAVE TWO BITES

You must continually convince yourself that you don't need to eat everything in sight. Statistics show that restaurants serve portions to fill a 180-pound man. For someone smaller than a big, bulky man to finish that portion is preposterous.

If we leave food control up the the body, we will never get fat. Always leave at least two bites of food on every plate, at every meal, every time. Force the body to exercise judgment about how much is enough. Grow accustomed to seeing food left behind; it will give you the freedom to get more if you are still hungry and the satisfaction of trusting your body to keep you thin and healthy.

Leaving food behind is especially important for those who are overweight and for those who have a food addiction. If you have ever polished off a box of cookies in one sitting, or an entire quart of ice cream, or a whole pizza, you have an eating problem. It may not be serious enough to make you fat right now, but it is the seed of a big problem. Leaving at least two bites of food behind every time you eat will check that problem for you at this point in its development. This simple habit, developed now, may save you from a nightmare later on.

MAKE IT A MEAL

If you are hungry and are going to permit yourself to eat in between your meals or after your dinner, make that food you prepare another meal, complete with all the rules and procedures you follow at all your other meals. The most important element when allowing yourself extra food is to eliminate the panic of eating and the guilt that follows. You can systematically eliminate panic, and perhaps the extra food, completely. Arrange the food on a special plate, preparing it as attractively as you can, and take it to a designated eating place. Relax and enjoy the food by taking small bites. Taste every morsel of your tempting treat. If you are going to eat, make it worthwhile. Enjoy everything that you eat, or don't eat it at all.

MAKE EATING IMPORTANT

Become a gourmet. Gourmets, people who love good food, are not fat. Fat people actually hate food. All addicted people hate the substance they are addicted to. You hate the things you fear, and fat people fear and hate food.

Recall how differently you feel when you are all dressed up, enjoying a meal in an elegant restaurant, from when you are sitting around a cluttered kitchen table in your old clothes eating mundane, unattractive food. There is quite a difference in your attitude and quite a difference in how you eat and how much you eat. The more elegant and fancy you feel when you eat, the more respect you give the food and the more satisfied you will be with less of it.

At home, set the prettiest table that you can. Never use paper napkins. Always use pretty cloth napkins. Use tablecloths or place mats and candles. Prepare yourself for eating. You don't have to be fancy to feel elegant. Just clean up, change your clothes, and perhaps put on some cologne. A pleasant fragrance is nice before you eat; it quiets the appetite and makes you feel very special.

Develop pleasure in eating. If you spend 30 minutes on each of your meals, you will experience taste sensations that you never knew before. Explore those food messages. Close your eyes and chew each bite of food slowly. Feel how the taste changes as food is ready to be swallowed. What does the texture feel like? How long does the taste last? Does the taste change as you chew? Experience the food that you are eating. You may find that some of the foods you thought you liked best really don't excite you the way you thought they did. Become intimate with food to control your eating, and you will eat everything you want without ever gaining weight.

BANK CALORIES

Everyone who controls his weight is aware of whether food is high or low in calories before he eats it. You must keep a quiet, ongoing tally of the number of calories that you consume and learn to bank calories to spend later on a special high-calorie meal.

Food combining will automatically trim calories from almost all of your meals. But beyond that you must keep your eyes open for every opportunity to eliminate unnecessary calories. Don't attempt to eliminate your favorite foods because they are caloric. That is food manipulation and will eventually make you fat. Enjoy your favorite foods, controlling when you eat them. Bank enough calories during the day to afford the cost.

For example, a glass of wine before dinner has approximately 100 calories. If you mix half wine and half soda water you will have a wonderful drink called a wine spritzer at half the cost in calories. How about this one? (It's my favorite.) Instead of cooking pasta, if you are in the mood for Italian food, steam up a big pot of fresh bean sprouts. They will take about 10 minutes to become soft and spaghettilike. Then pour your homemade spaghetti sauce over a plate of hot, steamed sprouts for the most wonderful "pasta" you have ever had and save a few hundred calories for something that really makes a difference. Also keep your eye on butter. It is high in calories and often goes untasted on many foods. I have even found that good French bread in a restaurant is just as good without butter than with it, and I am able to bank 40 or 50 calories with each slice.

NEVER SKIP BREAKFAST OR LUNCH

You will never control your eating if your blood sugar levels drastically fluctuate from spacing meals too far apart. Skipping breakfast or lunch will knock your blood sugar level for a loop and cause a condition of hypoglycemia that will be further aggravated by raising your blood sugar abruptly with a large dinner before retiring.

Your blood sugar level must be established as soon as you awaken in the morning. A breakfast of fruit will do that nicely as long as you eat lunch within four hours. Lunch is very important. It will boost your failing blood sugar level, and most important, it will keep you from those deadly late afternoon lows that drive you to sugar or coffee.

Low blood sugar stresses the body. The stress responses and the behavior related to this biochemical adjustment are involved in overeating and overdrinking. The results of low blood sugar can be devastating.

DON'T EAT FOR 30 MINUTES AFTER A MEAL

The momentum of eating can carry over for up to 30 minutes after finishing a meal. Food is stimulating, as you know, and the physical excitement of eating doesn't stop as soon as you feel full and finish eating. It may carry on and continue to stimulate. If eating after finishing a meal is your pattern, knowing why you continue to pick and snack after eating a full meal gives you the opportunity to put an end to that dangerous habit.

Remember that food is addicting, especially starch and protein. Continuing to eat after finishing a meal is a sign that addiction may be taking root. Without being conscious of it, you are allowing the stimulus of eating to become more important than it should be. To reverse that drive, make it a rule to wait 30 minutes after eating before you consider eating anything else, even dessert.

After 30 minutes the stimulating effect of eating will have faded and you will be able to determine more accurately whether or not more food is necessary. You may find that even the dessert that you had been anticipating will not be tempting after 30 minutes of cool-down.

WEIGH EVERY MORNING

You don't need a scale to tell you if you are gaining or losing. You will feel it. But the scale is a good tool for estimating how involved you may permit yourself to be with food that day.

If you see that the scale is registering above your acceptable weight level, you will want to handle food carefully all day, banking calories whenever you can and postponing that big dinner that you have been longing for until the next day. Just seeing the scale move above the ideal mark is enough to divert your interest in food for the day. This way, weight fluctuations are handled immediately, and you will never be shocked to find that you weigh five or six pounds more than you expected, which may drive you into dieting.

Conversely, if you find that you are on the light side of your mark, you may give yourself a green light should a dinner invitation tempt you.

If your weight seldom fluctuates, morning weighing is not important for you. But if your weight creeps up on you every now and again, as it does with most of us mortals, don't skip the morning weigh-in. Spot the trends before they become patterns.

ANTICIPATE; PLAN AHEAD

Never go into an eating situation without anticipating what you expect to find or without a plan for what you expect to eat. If you are going out to dinner, before you get to the restaurant, try to be familiar with what the restaurant has to offer and plan whether you will have protein or starch before you even get there.

Change your plan if something looks irresistible to you once you get to the dinner. That's perfectly OK. But just having a plan will keep you thinking and in control most of the time, saving you from the fat monster, who can creep up so easily when you are having fun.

RESTRICT CAFFEINE

Besides being enervated, caffeine is a drug that attacks your blood sugar, sending it soaring above normal limits before it comes crashing down to make you irritable, depressed, and hungry.

Coffee or tea will take the edge off hunger for a half hour or so, but most people don't realize that caffeine will make you hungry and will drive you to unwholesome food to find satisfaction.

LOOK AT YOURSELF DISROBED

Every day without fail, look at yourself disrobed in a full-length mirror. Know your body. Examine it from every side to know exactly what you look like. If you gain only two pounds, you will see it immediately, as long as you look at your body every day. Feeling extra weight, being heavy according to the scale, and then seeing your body a little fuller will all help keep you an arm's distance from food.

Many people have never examined themselves naked. Somewhere we were mistakenly taught not to look at the naked body, even our own. Discard that inhibition. If you want to achieve superior health, you must know everything that you can about yourself. Examining your body every day is as important to your attitude as exercise is for your muscles. Everyone in good shape knows what his body looks like and is proud to see it naked. If you don't like what you see right now, you will know exactly what to work on.

EXPECT FOOD DAYS

Everyone has days when the appetite is unreasonable and no amount of food will satisfy. No one knows where these food days come from, but they are common. If you have a weight problem, food days can frighten you, and being frightened can cause you to eat more than you would if you expected them.

Handle food days by eating more at meals if you must, but absolutely do not allow yourself to eat whenever or wherever food crosses your mind. Allow yourself the extra food, but tighten up on the rules that control your eating.

DO NOT FAST TO LOSE WEIGHT

You will regain every pound that you lose by fasting. Don't make the mistake of trying to lose weight by withholding food, even for one day.

This will be good news for those of you who can't afford to lose weight and want to fast to detoxify. Any weight that you lost during a cleansing fast will return as soon as you begin eating again. So don't avoid fasting: the weight loss is only temporary.

THE 10-PERCENT INVESTMENT

Weight control is a management problem. It is an investment proposition. Think of a trim body and superior health as rewards for investing only 10 percent of your time. If you could get nine to-one odds and be guaranteed a win, you would be in a new business without a moment's hesitation. So, if you invest just 2½ hours a day in your health and fitness, you will walk high for the rest of the 24 hours.

Think of it as an investment. Invest a half hour in each of your three properly combined meals and invest the other hour every day in exercise and personal grooming. For that pleasurable, small investment, you will ensure your best health—guaranteed!

Feel free to neglect the investment every once in awhile. You can afford to skip the exercise one day a week, and you can afford to miscombine a meal every so often without losing too much ground. You are the judge of how often and when. But keep in mind that it is a lot easier to maintain the edge than it is to regain it, once lost.

THREE WEEKS TO BUILD HABITS

Habits develop easily. You have heard it said that we are creatures of habit, and this is true. Most of the habits that own us were developed without our knowledge. They were established with repetition, and they won't disappear.

We can learn automatic behavior just as easily. As a matter of fact, the habits that we learn deliberately can be the strongest of all if they are planned properly and practiced long enough.

It is generally accepted that behavior can become automatic if it is repeated without deviation 21 consecutive times. If, after trying these weight control suggestions, you decide that some of them work well for you, repeat those behaviors for 21 days without changing their pattern, and you will build a dependable habit.

Sitting down to eat is a behavior that will serve everyone well. If you take your food to the table and sit down to eat it for the next 21 times that you are tempted to eat standing on your feet, you will erase the very thought of eating while you stand, and you will save five to 10 pounds a year. That's all there is to it.

The same procedure is effective in disassembling a habit. If you come home every day and go right to the kitchen for something to eat, practice substituting something else that can occupy your thoughts for 10–15 minutes as soon as you get home, for the next 21 days. The habit will be choked off. It may cross your mind every once in awhile for a spell, but the drive will be extinguished.

FOUR INCHES FROM LIPS TO SWALLOW

In the continual effort to control weight, there are times when we have to remind ourselves that there are only four inches from the lips to the swallow. That is a rather short distance of taste-pleasure to risk the misery of being fat—a very cheap thrill for a very long punishment.

10

Making It Work

Food combining is a discipline that can be practiced success-fully all the time and in all situations. First, however, it must be experienced and practiced long enough to provide rewards that are more important than the temptation to miscombine.

In other words, food combining will become a part of your life, and must become a part of your life, if you give it a chance. Food combining must be learned and practiced before it will stand the test of dinner parties, vacations, holidays, and other eating occasions.

By now you have properly combined a few meals and have felt better or at least different. You probably have also found it difficult at times to combine properly the food that was forced on you or was served at expensive restaurants. If so, you are now on the way to "making it work" so that you may become healthier, live longer, and combine food properly for the rest of your life. Be determined to take time, effort, and thought to make food combining work for you.

THE THREE-WEEK PLAN

It takes three weeks, or 21 repetitions, of a new behavior to establish a habit pattern. If you don't make a habit of food combining (and exercising, too) you will only enjoy benefits when little effort is involved and you will never achieve the full health potential that food combining can provide. It is up to you. To find out how easily food combining and aerobics can be healthy parts of your lifestyle, take the next three weeks to work at self-improvement. You have nothing to lose, except perhaps some weight.

For the next three weeks, make food combining the first consideration when you plan your meals. It is easy. You will find that only a few meals will need major restructuring because most combinations are made acceptable with only minor adjustments. It just takes some planning. Do not miss this opportunity to improve your health and to control more of your life.

SHORT-TERM GOALS

Succeeding at anything requires setting goals. Goals set too far into the future don't supply the rewards along the way that help you sustain continuous effort. They invite boredom, discouragement, and then failure. To incorporate food combining into your lifestyle you must proceed from one meal to the next and from one day to the next. Look no further ahead than tomorrow. Each meal will reward you with a delightful feeling of well-being, and each day will bring you success and confidence.

BEGIN WITH A PLAN

The next three weeks will permanently place food combining among the more preferred rituals in your life. Decide exactly when you will begin this training. Have a plan; do not leave it up to chance. The weekend is a good time to begin food combining. Routine pressures are off, and your meals may be addressed in leisurely fashion. Or Monday morning may be a good time to begin something new. Find the best time for you. Although you will be working from one meal to the next, for the first week of the three-week training period you should plan to be especially exact, working carefully to lay a sturdy foundation on which to build. And start when you can foresee a relatively uncluttered week. The first week is the most important.

You are trying to change a behavior pattern, not your taste in food. The behavior of haphazardly mixing different foods together at the same time is about to be examined and changed. Make it easy on yourself. For the first week, stay away from eating situations that are not within your control. Do not tempt yourself with food that is poorly combined until you develop the preference for not wanting it, and you most definitely will. Give yourself every opportunity to experience the rewards of food combining. Guard against reinforcing old thoughtless combinations of food; intermittent reinforcement of old behavior builds the strongest ties to that behavior. Take this project on with enthusiasm. A part-time effort will miss the target.

SHARING

You will find that the experience of food combining will make a more permanent impression on you if you begin with a friend. So many unbelievable changes will happen to you after beginning to food-combine that you will want someone to share them with.

On the other side of the coin, be prepared for resistance from members of your family who are not using food combining. For some strange reason, friends and loved ones will frequently sabotage your plans for self-improvement that they don't share. Try to include your family and friends in your new food combining program, but if they show no interest, expect them to trip you when they can.

KEEP A JOURNAL

Why not keep a record of your experience? Food combining may turn out to be the most significant improvement you have ever made in your health. Keeping a journal of your first three weeks will increase your involvement and will help you to understand the improvements that you make. Record everything that you eat, how long it took you to eat it, and your mood and attitude about food combining at the time. You may discover things about yourself that will surprise you. You may learn, for instance, that you feel deprived and sorry for yourself when you try to eliminate toast from your morning egg meal, perhaps even angry and irritable for the rest of the morning. An insight like that can help to put your thinking in order and organize your efforts.

Whatever keeping a journal highlights for you, it is interesting and fun and certain to teach you more about food combining.

BREAKFAST

Things to Remember

If you are accustomed to having a hearty breakfast, this meal may prove to be the most difficult to combine properly. Our custom of having fruit, protein, and starch at breakfast is so entrenched that it can be a problem to eliminate part of the meal without feeling that it is incomplete. You may find yourself craving the missing part of the usual breakfast. Don't fall for it, though. Tell yourself that for lunch you will have all the toast that you want, so postpone until later those parts of the meal that don't combine well now.

How to Make It Work

1. Do not skip breakfast. Low blood sugar causes depression.
2. Switch to an all-fruit breakfast. That is best for cleansing and energizing.
3. Combine the following.
   - Hot cereal with butter and/or cream
   - Cold cereal with cream
   - Toast, bagel, muffin with butter
4. Do not combine the following.
   - Eggs with toast, bagel, muffin
   - Eggs with potatoes
   - Toast, bagel, muffin with jams, jellies, cream cheese, or peanut butter
   - Fruit with cereal or protein

- Protein with protein
- Fruit or fruit juice with protein or starch

5. Realize that no one's feelings are more important than your health. Assert yourself.

LUNCH

Things to Remember

Lunch is the easiest meal to combine properly and may just be the pivotal meal of the day. Don't skip it.

Blood sugar falls rapidly four or five hours after a meal. If left unchecked, low blood sugar impairs thinking, causes fatigue and irritability, ruins concentration, and dims eyesight. Without lunch, you will make more mistakes during the afternoon and be more confused and anxious.

Lunch is easiest to combine properly in a restaurant, where you can order exactly what you want to eat. Decide before you eat whether you will have a protein, starch, or fruit meal. If you begin with the bread that the waiter puts on the table, continue throughout the meal with starch and vegetables. If your plan is to order a protein meal, tell the waiter not to bring bread. If it isn't there on the table, you will not even think of it.

Salads should dominate lunch. Protein is more stimulating than starch. Starch can be somewhat sleep-inducing for many people and may be a better choice for your evening meal. All sandwiches are poor combinations except for avocado sandwiches or sandwiches made with vegetables other than tomatoes. And beware of the salad dressing. Restaurant and commercially made dressings usually contain sugar, stabilizers, and vinegar.

How to Make It Work

1. Do not skip lunch. It may be the most important meal, since blood sugar falling from breakfast can turn into an emergency by dinner.
2. Stay with fruit (like breakfast). If so, do not combine fruit with anything else.

3. Brown-baggers may take cottage cheese, yogurt, cheese and fruit, salad, vegetable sandwiches.

4. Realize that no one's feeling are more important than your health. Assert yourself.

DINNER

Things to Remember

Dinner is the least important meal of the day with regard to the body's need for nutrients and the ability of the digestive system to process and to eliminate efficiently. During sleep the metabolism is slowed down as much as 25 percent. A dinner meal high in protein, eaten before retiring, will keep the blood sugar level elevated high enough to interfere with sleep, and food may be delayed in the stomach as long as eight hours, awaiting full digestive power. A starch meal may not delay sleep but will surely be digested slowly by the resting metabolism and may produce gas and discomfort that will affect your next day's performance.

Let salads and vegetables dominate the last meal of the day. Of course, dinner at home will be the easiest to combine properly. But restaurants present no obstacle to food combining unless you don't speak up about what you want. And dinner parties will ruin your good intentions unless you arrive prepared to follow your plan of eating either protein or starch. Also, don't permit yourself to eat while standing and wait a full half hour after dinner before entertaining any thought of dessert. Your first few dinner parties and restaurant outings will be the toughest. During the three-week break-in, do your best to stay away from temptations that encourage miscombining and overeating. Face those tough tests after you have some history of success with lesser battles and be prepared to tackle the first few trials with a solid plan and a stiff upper lip.

How to Make It Work

1. Drink alcohol before dinner, if you must. It is not best while eating.

2. Plan ahead for restaurants and parties.
3. Decide on protein or starch before you eat. Consider your last two meals before deciding.
4. Include a raw vegetable salad in all your dinners for a healthy digestive system.
5. Follow a heavy dinner with a fresh fruit breakfast.

SNACKS

Things to Remember

Most snacking is done in response to external eating cues like a certain time of day, a coffee break, returning home, seeing food, smelling food, etc. Feeling hunger in between your meals indicates poor meal planning and may require the addition of another meal to raise your blood sugar. Make all snacks official meals, complete with all the rules of civilized eating mentioned earlier. Carefully select snacks that don't interfere with the digestion of the previous and the following meals.

Snacking is the major cause of overweight. Making a meal of snacks will help to eliminate unnecessary eating in between meals by making it more difficult to plan and to execute.

How to Make It Work

1. Do not snack on your feet—*a must!*
2. Eat fruit in the afternoon but not after a protein lunch.
3. Eat sugar snacks alone, well before or after meals.
4. Don't drink coffee or drink it black.

HOLIDAYS

Things to Remember

Unless you are dedicated to food combining and the continual improvement of your health, family holiday eating will always give you trouble.

The best approach to holiday eating may just be to prepare for inevitable miscombining with meals of fresh fruit and raw salads before and after the festivities.

Two days before Thanksgiving or Christmas dinner, eat mainly raw vegetable salads, little protein and starch, and high-fiber fruit like pineapple or papaya on the morning of the dinner. When you get to dinner, try to combine properly by eating either the protein, like turkey or ham, and the vegetables, or forego the protein to eat the starch dressing, potatoes, vegetables, etc. You are bound to miscombine by eating more than one starch or one protein at the meal. But by deciding on either protein or starch you will at least eliminate the most offensive miscombination. Eating slowly is very important at a meal with such a variety of food. Overeating and miscombining at the same meal produce immediate and long-term stress that can be damaging. So, if you choose to miscombine, space the incompatible foods far apart, eat slowly, and listen carefully to your appestat signal to stop. It may help to remember before you eat how uncomfortable you were last year after the same dinner.

As with all miscombined meals, follow the holiday eating with a large fresh fruit breakfast and raw vegetable salads for the next two meals to unclog the digestive system and to contribute alkalinity to the blood made more acid by overeating.

How to Make It Work

1. Arrive well fed. Missed meals before banquets result in overeating.
2. Combine one holiday meal properly and you may never miscombine again.
3. Wait as long as you can before having dessert.
4. Eat protein first and then starch if you must miscombine.
5. Eat slowly. Less damage is done.

TRAVEL

Things to Remember

Food combining while traveling is easy as long as you are not trapped someplace where you are forced to eat inferior food. You can order vegetarian meals on all air flights if you inform the airline a day or two before. You will be delighted with the freshness of a special-order meal on an airplane.

Always order your own food. Don't allow tour guides or friends or relatives to order for you. If there is special food to be tested, find out what it is so you may coordinate the other foods in the meal. Properly combined food will also minimize your chances of becoming constipated and getting sick—two things that can spoil your travel plans.

Cruise ships and resorts that include food spell trouble. Vacations like these tempt gluttonous eaters to eat everything. If that is your interest, you have already made your plan; but if you travel for other reasons, stay away or stay very busy.

Time off from work is not time off from healthy eating and exercise. Insist on food combining while traveling and fit in at least a little daily exercise, both of which will allow you to enjoy yourself more and to return home without excess weight and guilt. No matter where you go, don't mix protein, starch, or sugar at the same meal and at least run in place for 20 minutes in your hotel room, if you must, every day. Ensure your good health with the high cost of travel.

How to Make It Work

1. Order special meals on airplanes.
2. Bring dried fruit and nuts for emergencies.
3. Eat a lot of fruit and raw vegetables often. They are nonconstipating.
4. Continue to exercise. You will feel better and eat less.
5. Order your own food. Insist on it.

EXERCISE

Things to Remember

The proper beginning of an exercise program determines your success at maintaining it. Plan three weeks of slow development before realizing any rewards. Let your heart rate guide your speed and progress and your good judgment keep your nose to the wheel. Exercise may not always be fun, but the results are spectacular. If you are waiting to lose some weight or to feel better or to be in a better frame of mind to enjoy exercise, it is time to abandon that foolish notion. Exercise is somewhat like medicine. Decision makes it easy on you. Learn to exercise right so that the rewards stay ahead of the pain.

The most beneficial schedule for exercising is to do some kind of aerobic movement every day, alternating exercises each day to give specific muscles time off to repair and to grow stronger. It is very important that you plan a regular time each day to be reserved for exercise. Exercise only three times the first week, but reserve the time to be used each day. If you don't establish a regular schedule, you will not develop the habit of exercising. Even if you don't use the time to exercise, separate it from the rest of the day so that it will always cue you.

How to Make It Work

1. Begin aerobic exercise slowly—12 minutes at your training heart rate, three times the first week.
2. Reserve the same time every day for your body—the only way to develop a habit is to repeat it.
3. Develop at least two alternating aerobic exercises—one for inside, one for outside. This prevents soreness and boredom and makes exercising every day possible.
4. Do your own thing, though company helps motivate you.
5. Do not exceed your training heart rate. Be able to carry on a conversation, for instance.
6. Use the best equipment that you can find. It makes a big difference in your enthusiasm and your progress.

THE LAST WORD

Remember, this information is intended for people who want to know more about being healthy. It is for those people who want to achieve and maintain a sound mind and a body that works at peak efficiency throughout a longer life.

11

Meal Planning—Getting Started

The following meal plans will illustrate properly combined meals. While they may be followed exactly, they are offered as examples of proper food combining with regard to digestive capability as well as the proper balance of alkaline/acid and raw/cooked foods.

Summer/spring and winter/fall menus have been differentiated primarily because of the extra heat that must be generated from food to keep the body warmer during cold weather.

During the winter, when fresh fruit is not always available in great variety and at reasonable cost, some substituting may be necessary. Whole-grain cereal or stone-ground, whole-grain toast can replace fruit for breakfast during the winter months. When substituting, remember to replace fruit breakfast with other high-fiber foods. Adding bran flakes to your cereal is always good insurance.

If you want to excel in preparing properly combined and highly creative meals, ask your bookstore to order *Cooking Naturally,* by John Calella, published by And/Or Press, Berkeley, California. His recipes are challenging and wonderful. The two that follow are typical and are sure to pique the taste of everyone with more than a passing interest in food.

ASPARAGUS AND MUSHROOM SAUCE

Ingredients

1½ lbs. asparagus
2 oz. olive oil
1 oz. water
1 oz. mineral bouillon
1½ lbs. mushrooms

1 bunch parsley, chopped
2 stalks celery, chopped
2 cloves garlic, chopped
2 oz. mineral bouillon
2 oz. olive oil

Cut asparagus stalks in half; sauté bottom halves in 2 oz. olive oil, 1 oz. water, and 1 oz. mineral bouillon for 10–12 minutes. Drain stock into a small bowl and blend sautéed asparagus ends in blender. Combine in a small mixing bowl the mushrooms, parsley, celery, garlic, 2 oz. mineral bouillon, 2 oz. olive oil, and the stock from the sautéed asparagus ends. Combine the asparagus ends in blender and blend into a creamy thick sauce. Place asparagus tips on a serving platter and cover with the mushroom-asparagus sauce. Broil for 3–5 minutes. Serve.

BRUSSELS SPROUTS

Ingredients

2 red onions, chopped
3 oz. water
2 oz. olive oil
1 oz. mineral bouillon
2 T. mineral powder
2 lbs. Brussels sprouts

½ head cabbage, finely chopped
5 carrots, diced
2 russet potatoes, diced
2 oz. olive oil
1 oz. water

Preheat oven at 450° F. for 10 minutes. Prepare an onion sauce: Put chopped onions into a covered roasting pan with 3 oz. water, 2 oz. olive oil, 1 oz. mineral bouillon, and 2 tablespoons mineral powder. Reduce oven to 350° F. and bake onions for 3 minutes. While onion sauce is cooking, trim Brussels sprouts, removing stems and any blemished leaves. Add Brussels sprouts and chopped cabbage to the onion sauce and bake for another 5–8minutes. Meanwhile, sauté diced carrots and potatoes in 2 oz. olive oil and 1 oz. water for 5 to 8 minutes. Remove Brussels sprouts and cabbage from oven and place in a large serving dish. Cover with sautéed vegetables, and serve.

ONE-WEEK MEAL PLAN
WINTER/FALL

Breakfast	*Lunch*	*Dinner*
Monday		
Bananas and cream	Vegetable salad	Baked potato stuffed with sautéed onions or with butter and sour cream
	Tuna fish	
		Two cooked nonstarchy vegetables
		Vegetable salad
Tuesday		
Oatmeal with butter and cinnamon	Vegetable salad	Lentil soup
	Mushroom omelette (no bread)	Whole-wheat bread with butter
		Vegetable salad
Wednesday		
Papaya	Avocado sandwich with bacon	Fresh broiled fish
Oranges		Two nonstarchy vegetables
		Vegetable salad
Thursday		
Grapefruit	Vegetable salad with chicken or turkey	Baked yam with butter, sour cream, and chives
Slice of hard cheese		Vegetable salad

Friday

Stewed prunes	Yogurt, plain	Spaghetti with marinara sauce
Buttermilk or kefir	Oranges or grapefruit	Vegetable salad

Saturday

Pineapple	Vegetable salad with nuts, seeds, and raisins	Baked eggplant or vegetable casserole with French garlic bread

Sunday

Apples	Hamburger patty with onions	Sautéed Oriental vegetables served over steamed rice
Grapes	Vegetable salad	
Dried Fruit		

ONE-WEEK MEAL PLAN
SUMMER/SPRING

Breakfast	*Lunch*	*Dinner*
Monday		
Cantaloupe	Apples	Fresh corn on the cob with melted butter
	Hard cheese	Vegetable salad
Tuesday		
Prunes	Citrus fruit	Baked acorn squash with butter and cinnamon
Apricots	Cottage cheese	Vegetable salad

Wednesday

Fresh berries with cream	Yogurt with fresh fruit	Broiled or baked chicken
		Vegetable salad

Thursday

Watermelon	Vegetable salad with cottage cheese	Vegetable salad with avocado
		Dark bread with butter

Friday

Honeydew melon	Chef salad	Baked potato with sautéed onions or butter and sour cream
		Vegetable salad

Saturday

Peaches	Cashew nuts with fresh strawberries	Spinach or avocado pasta with oil and garlic
Plums		Vegetable salad

Sunday

Mango	Omelette with sautéed onions and peppers	Wild rice with sautéed onions and mushrooms
Cherries		Vegetable salad

During the summer and spring, when fresh fruit is abundant, vary your breakfast every day with fruit that is in the height of season each week. You can easily determine which fruit is currently most available by following the prices in the market and buying when prices drop.

A relaxing Sunday at home is an excellent opportunity to clean out your system and enjoy the wonderful pleasure of eating nothing but fruit all day. After a day of eating all fruit, you will find that you will be more thoughtful about your selection of food for the rest of the week.

The meal plans are intended to guide you during the first week. After that, begin to experiment. Fresh vegetable juice can replace fruit or be added before or after any meal. Sauces can be made for any dish. Dishes that are normally served hot may be just as good chilled—chilled pasta dishes, for instance, are famous and delicious. Steamed bean sprouts make a very interesting substitute for spaghetti—just steam 1½ or 2 pounds of sprouts until they are wilted. Let them drain, arrange them as you would spaghetti on a plate hot from the oven, and pour marinara or meat sauce over them. This serves two people. Serve with garlic bread. The possibilities of preparing interesting and wholesome meals without miscombining are endless. Any health food store will have dozens of cookbooks that hundreds of exceptional meals can be taken from.

If you have no special interest in cooking, your variations on the suggested menus may be few. Make a point, however, to alter your selection of foods continually, especially protein. Each food provides something that is a little different. A large variety of food will keep us the healthiest.

Index